*Medicine & Society
In America*

Medicine & Society
In America

Advisory Editor

Charles E. Rosenberg
Professor of History
University of Pennsylvania

THE

CAUSATION, COURSE, AND TREATMENT

OF

REFLEX INSANITY IN WOMEN

BY

HORATIO ROBINSON STORER, M.D., LL.B.

ARNO PRESS & THE NEW YORK TIMES
New York   1972

Reprint Edition 1972 by Arno Press Inc.

Reprinted from a copy in
The Library of The College of
Physicians of Philadelphia

LC# 71-180592
ISBN 0-405-03974-3

Medicine and Society in America
ISBN for complete set: 0-405-03930-1
See last pages of this volume for titles.

Manufactured in the United States of America

THE

CAUSATION, COURSE, AND TREATMENT

OF

REFLEX INSANITY IN WOMEN.

BY

HORATIO ROBINSON STORER, M. D., LL. B.,

OF BOSTON,

Surgeon to St. Elizabeth's and St. Francis's Hospitals for Women ; Consulting Surgeon to the Carney (General) Hospital ; formerly Assistant in Obstetrics and Medical Jurisprudence in Harvard University, Professor of Obstetrics and the Diseases of Women in Berkshire Medical College, and Physician to the Boston Lying-in-Hospital ; late Vice-President of the American Medical Association ; Member of the Gynæcological Society of Boston, the New York Medico-Legal Society, the Obstetric and Medico-Chirurgical Societies of Edinburgh ; Corresponding Member of the Obstetrical Society of Berlin ; Honorary Member of the Louisville Obstetrical Society, and of the Canadian Medical Association.

Sublatâ causâ, tollitur effectus.

BOSTON:
LEE AND SHEPARD, PUBLISHERS.
NEW YORK:
LEE, SHEPARD AND DILLINGHAM.
1871.

Entered, according to Act of Congress, in the year 1870,
BY LEE AND SHEPARD,
In the Office of the Librarian of Congress, at Washington.

STEREOTYPED AT THE
BOSTON STEREOTYPE FOUNDRY,
19 Spring Lane.

TO THE

MEMBERS OF THE GYNÆCOLOGICAL SOCIETY
OF BOSTON,

THOUGHTFUL, WORKING, FEARLESS GENTLEMEN,

ALREADY A POWER IN THE LAND,

This Book

IS AFFECTIONATELY INSCRIBED.

PREFATORY NOTE.

THE following pages were communicated to the American Medical Association in 1865, at its session in Boston, and were printed in its Transactions for that year. The writer has been requested to republish his memoir by physicians interested in gynæcology, who have desired a copy in a separate form for their book-shelves, or have thought the topic deserving more general attention; and he was duly authorized to do so by a formal vote of the Association,* at its session at Cincinnati in 1867.

Many causes have combined to prevent accedence to the wish of his friends and the repeated request of his publishers, chief among them, perhaps, the feeling that, as he had sown the seed, it should be for others to develop the tender growth of a better practice. He has cherished the lingering hope, moreover, that he might some time find leisure to prepare a work upon this interesting subject of reflex insanity more worthy its intrinsic and practical importance.

That leisure, however, has not yet arrived; and the publication by Professor Louis Mayer, of Berlin, in the last volume of the Transactions of the Obstetrical Society of that city, of an elaborate paper upon the relations of the fe-

---

* Transactions of the Association, vol. xviii., 1867, p. 43. By its constitution, all scientific communications made to the Association become its exclusive property, and cannot be published by their authors without express permission.

male sexual organs to mental disease, has seemed to afford a suitable moment for simultaneously presenting the two memoirs to the medical public in this country.* It will be perceived that, approaching the subject from a somewhat different stand-point, and in entire ignorance that he had been anticipated in the investigation by several years, Professor Mayer affords unanswerable proof of the correctness of every point made in the following pages.

The writer has preferred, in view of his inability to revise and extend the paper, to make no material changes in it whatsoever.

HOTEL PELHAM, BOSTON, 1 November, 1870.

* A translation of Prof. Mayer's memoir, by Dr. George H. Bixby, with notes by Dr. Storer, will be found in the Journal of the Gynæcological Society of Boston, commencing with the number for May, 1870. Discussions upon the general subject of insanity in women have been held at several of the meetings of the Society, reports of which have also been published in its Journal.

CONTENTS.

		PAGE
I.	Selection of Special Topic.	9
II.	Point previously attained.	21
III.	Work to be done..	30
IV.	The Brain the Seat of Insanity, not always of its Cause..	36
V.	Explanations of distant Causation.	62
VI.	Causation of Insanity often Pelvic in Women.	77
VII.	Rationale of Pelvic Causation of Insanity.	127
VIII.	Indications of Treatment.	157

THE CAUSATION, COURSE, AND TREATMENT OF REFLEX INSANITY IN WOMEN.

I.—Selection of special Topic.

It was decided at the meeting of the American Medical Association, held at St. Louis, in 1854, to establish a standing committee, annually to be chosen, and regularly to report " upon the subject of insanity as it prevails in this country, including its causation, as hereditary transmission, educational influences,—physical and moral,—social and political institutions, &c.; its forms and complications, curability, means of prevention, &c."

In 1865, eleven years had elapsed since the committee was first appointed, and to that time there seems to have been rendered no report. Special committees, it is true, upon particular points, selected by the Association, and connected with the general subject of insanity, had twice attended to the duties assigned to them, preparing the excellent papers upon the Medical Jurisprudence of Insanity, by Dr. Coventry, of Utica, N. Y., and upon Moral Insanity in its Relations to Medical Jurisprudence, by the late

Dr. D. Meredith Reese, of New York city,— both of them rendered to the meeting held at Washington in 1858, and contained in the published volume of the Transactions of the Association for that year. A similar report upon the Morbid and Therapeutical Effects of Mental and Moral Influences had been promised by Professor Palmer, of Michigan. As regards, however, the regular standing committee upon insanity, the fact remains as stated: it had uniformly failed to accomplish its work.*

This is the more surprising when we consider to what extent the subject had already been studied in this country, the excellence to which our general system of hospital arrangement had been brought, and the eminence attained by many American superintendents.

These gentlemen had been freely placed upon the committee appointed by the Association in years past, if not, indeed, in each previous instance selected from them alone, and it is a matter of extreme regret that they should not have responded to the call; for there are few subjects attended with the interest to

---

* Dr. Hills, of Ohio, at that time superintendent of the Central Lunatic Asylum at Columbus, who was charged with the duty of reporting at the New York meeting, as chairman of the committee on insanity for 1864, was prevented from fulfilling that trust; among other causes, by "the breadth of foundation he had laid for an elaborate report." At his request, he was granted an extension of time. with the understanding, however, that this arrangement did not interfere with the appointment of the new committee for 1865, which it was understood by the nominating committee was then annually required by the organic law of the Association.

the profession at large that pertains to this of insanity; few with such important bearings upon the welfare of the community, and its relations to medical men, — few with such fruitful fields for labor and success.

It will undoubtedly be alleged, that in the fact that the hospital superintendents of the several States had united themselves into a separate organization, — the so-called Association of Superintendents, meeting annually for purposes of conference, and publishing a journal devoted to the interests of their speciality, — there was enough accomplished for all the purposes of science and practical art, leaving it unnecessary for any annual contribution to either to be made through other channels. We, however, of the profession at large, can hardly acknowledge the justice of such reasoning. Special journals, however ably conducted, and with whatever extent of circulation, do not reach every general practitioner. As well ought it be said that any contribution to the science of ophthalmology — which, of all the departments of mediicine, now seems to boast the largest and most enthusiastic number of skilled devotees — would be out of place or undervalued with ourselves, simply because that branch has now its own national organization and its special journals.

Every specialist, no matter what his favorite study, whether insanity, ophthalmology, or the diseases of women, owes his first duty to the profession at large, for it is through it that his observations or his discoveries must really become effective. It is through those that apply upon the widest scale theories to practice, and practice to its ultimate demonstrations, that the largest results are to be gained; and, in this matter of insanity, for every patient that is carried to an asylum for treatment, scores are treated in their earlier stages, wherein the chances of success are allowed to be infinitely the greater, by the profession outside asylum walls; and for every patient that is ultimately cured in an asylum, in hundreds the derangement threatening is warded off by judicious general or special treatment at home, or in changed localities.

Now, be it distinctly understood that no man can put a higher value than I do upon our public hospitals for the insane. There are few of the profession, not directly connected with these institutions as physician or trustee, who have studied them more carefully, or upon a larger scale, both in their minute details and their comparative plans and methods of management. I believe them to be excellently conducted, and most of their medical officers to be men well selected, of skill, and worthy the highest trust. The records of the Association of these gentlemen show the most painstaking and extended efforts at improvement, and reflect, as does the Journal conducted in its behalf,* much credit upon itself collectively, and its individual members. Had, however, the Society of Superintendents but put itself into more direct connection with the General Association, of which its members were, and still are, almost every one of them in fellowship, it would have effected more towards establishing the high standard and accomplishing the good it has intended.

The opinion has prevailed in many quarters — it has, to a certain extent, been inculcated, as in the most excellent work upon the medical jurisprudence of insanity, by my friend, Dr. Isaac Ray — that no one can possibly know much of insanity, or at any rate be accepted as of any authority upon the subject, unless he is a member, as superintendent or ex-superintendent, of this inner circle.

But a man cannot study a special point in medicine with interest, assiduity, and good faith for many years, without forming decided conclusions thereon. If, moreover, his position, by accident or other advantage, has been such as to render him perfectly independent of all party or individual bias, *nullius addictus jurare in verba magistri*, these conclusions should have the greater weight; and if, in addition, he approaches the subject from a standpoint comparatively new, certainly so far as previous employment of it to attain a practical end has been concerned, and if he is able to show that measures which in one

---

* The American Journal of Insanity, Utica, N. Y.

quarter, namely, in civil practice, are found very effective for cure, in another quarter, namely, in asylum practice, are as yet generally and practically unrecognized, his conclusions should be very apt to carry with them conviction.

Such, I would respectfully submit, is my own position with regard to the present report. It is offered as a plain, straightforward statement of facts, commending themselves to the good sense of every member of the profession.

Upon the general subject of insanity volumes upon volumes have already been written, some of them of interest, and very practical use, much of them of none. I have no desire to add to the host of abstruse and abstract discussions of metaphysical points in psychology, already far too numerous. Were I an asylum superintendent, I might delight the Association by a discourse upon the excellent systems by which hospitals are now heated and ventilated, or the question as to whether, as regards economy, it is better for superintendents to raise or to purchase their own supplies; upon the psychological characteristics of Milton, Shakspeare, Dante, and the several *dramatis personæ*, supernal, mortal, or demoniac, of these and other writers; upon the comparative merits of restraint and non-restraint, and as to where the latter is supposed to begin and to end; whether Aubanel or Brigham invented the crib, and its advantages as compared with the bedstrap of Wyman, and this again with the fingerless gloves of Parkmann, the handless sleeves and muff of Haslam, the belts of Reil, and of the York Retreat, the manacles of Ruer, and the chains of time immemorial, the bifurcated sack of Horn, the knee breeches of Neumann, and the buckled straps of Nostitz, the leathern mask of Autenrieth, the pear-shaped frame for the mouth, and the gag, the wicker basket of Guislain, the suspended box of Hayner, the cord and the restraining chair, the dark chamber and the padded room, the rotary machine of Darwin, the suspended seat of Cox, the hanging mat of Hallaran, the hollow wheel of Hayner, the swing of Chiarruggi, the douche and the surprise bath, the proposal of our own Rush, whose treatise had for many years a more extensive circulation among American physicians than all other works upon mental disorders together, that because refractory horses are subdued by being kept from lying down or sleeping, and because elephants, when first captured, are tamed by depriving them of food until they discover signs of great emaciation, therefore the insane should be kept in a standing posture, and awake, for four and twenty hours, and fasting for several days!

These might be discussed, and other methods of subduing violent maniacs, and whether a little etherization is not, after all, much the best; upon whether, in insanity, the mind is or is not diseased, or is only partially hidden by a transient cloud; upon the pathological results of insanity, and why it is that in every affection of the mind, no matter how diverse or opposite, we may find identical conditions of the brain, or no trace of disease whatever, and in every lesion whatever of the brain we may find an entirely unaffected mind; and the host of other theoretical, practical, and transcendental questions so fully and so ably discussed in the pages of the American Journal of Insanity, of the Asylum Journal of Mental Science, of the Journal of Psychological Medicine, and the other periodicals devoted to the interests of the insane. As it is, having been chosen by the Association to this work in consequence, as I suppose, of having long been delving in the special field of hysteria, and the reflex nervous and neuralgic demonstrations of invalid women, I take it for granted that what is expected at my hands is, to a certain extent, of a special character, although of necessity, as all specialism rests upon general principles, I shall endeavor not to lose sight of the general basis upon which it lies.

The *causation* and the *cure* of insanity are its Alpha and Omega. The last of these has usually been sought the first; and it is because the other, upon which it wholly depends, is so often unsearched for wisely, if at all, that both are so seldom attained.

In deciding, therefore, to devote the major part of this report to an attempt at an elucidation of the true causation of mental disturbance in a large proportion of the cases in which it obtains in women, and of a more rational treatment than is generally adopted, I took early occasion to consult my colleagues upon the committee, who were all of them superintendents, and, without a single exception, of public and State hospitals for the insane. They were Drs. Bancroft, of New Hampshire; Van Deusen, of Michigan; Patterson, of Iowa; Woodburn, of Indiana; and Worthington, of the Friends' Asylum at Frankford, Pennsylvania.

With reference to the opinions of these gentlemen as expressed in letters from which I shall quote, it may be stated that I had previously avowed it as my belief that very many cases of mental disturbance in women are of reflex character, arising from pelvic irritation, and that local treatment would prove of advantage in very many more cases than those for which as yet it had ever been employed.

Dr. Bancroft wrote me as follows: —

"I freely admit that a large proportion of cases of insanity, even in both sexes, are of reflex origin, and not the result, primarily, of cerebral change.

"I am well aware, also, that many attacks of insanity in females originate in uterine disturbance of some sort, and are cured by treatment directed to that organ.

"A part of these cases, I have no doubt, require topical treatment, and, of course, demand examination by tact and the speculum. *No one would be more thankful than myself for better facilities than are at present afforded for investigating and teaching these cases.**

"What would be the best method of accomplishing this object, I have not yet a settled opinion.

"I have read your published articles in the Boston Medical and Surgical Journal;† and, if I correctly understand you, you hold that the principal cause of insanity in females is uterine disorder of some kind, and that the principal treatment in females is therefore to be directed to the uterus; and I infer further from your writings that topical treatment stands, or should stand, most prominent.

"Although admitting, to a more limited extent, the truth of your positions, yet I am not prepared to give that form of disease so prominent a place as to give to it the whole report, to the exclusion of other topics.

"Although your idea is one of importance, and should receive a due share of attention, I think to allow it to absorb the whole report would but partially and imperfectly discuss the great points of interest pertaining to insanity in this country."

From Dr. Worthington I received a communication of similar import.

"I believe it is the general opinion among asylum physicians," he said, "that insanity, in a great majority of cases, is unattended with any organic cerebral change; and the large number of cases of the disease attributable to ill health, in the reports of hospitals for the insane, is evidence of the belief of their authors that the disease is very commonly consecutive to disorders of the general system. Among these disorders, I have no doubt that those of the genital apparatus, in both sexes, are productive of a considerable number of cases of insanity. I can call to mind a

---

* The Italics above are my own, and are used because of the importance of the admission here made, in reference to incidental points hereafter to be considered.

† Loc. cit., April 7, October 13, and November 24, 1864.

case where a simple displacement of the uterus was the cause of an attack of insanity of two years' duration, which was remedied in this institution, in a short time, by confining the patient to bed, and applying a suitable pessary. In all cases under my care, where there is reason to believe that uterine disease may be the cause of the mental disorder, I have always been in the habit of making special examinations, and I have sometimes called in the assistance of medical friends who have made these diseases an especial study.

"On the other hand, I have gradually become convinced that we may attach too much importance to these disorders as a cause of insanity, and that in our willingness to refer the mental symptoms to irritation reflected from the uterus, we may overlook the more serious idiopathic cerebral disease. I have known the latter occur coincident with uterine disorder, and yet entirely independent of it; and have myself lost valuable time in treating the uterine affection, and afterwards, on addressing my remedies to the true seat of the mental disorder, have had the satisfaction of seeing my patient speedily recover. Such cases may not be very numerous, but they are very important to bear in mind, and I would beg leave to call your attention specially to them. It appears to me to be particularly desirable to discover in the character of the mental disorder itself, without reference to other symptoms, some marks by which we may be able to decide whether a case is one of idiopathic or sympathetic cerebral disorder."

Dr. Van Deusen confined himself to the discussion of a single point only, and that merely an incidental one as compared with the broad subject upon which I addressed him, and concerning which we have seen Drs. Bancroft and Worthington so fully expressing their opinion. The matter to which his communication is limited is that upon which I had read a paper at the previous meeting of the Association, which will be found published in the volume of its Transactions for 1864, namely, the necessity, for the more thorough elucidation of each case of insanity in females, that consulting physicians should be appointed to every hospital for the insane. To Dr. Van Deusen's letter I shall hereafter refer.

Dr. Woodburn wrote me as follows: —

"I read your articles, published some time since in the Boston Medical and Surgical Journal, and was well pleased with the contents; but would venture to suggest that probably insanity is not so frequently caused by female diseases as the papers would seem to indicate. My opinion is, that mental derangement is always caused, either by physical disease or bodily injury (accidental cases), or by malformation (hereditary cases). The malformation may be apparent, or may possibly be only of the elementary cells.

"I had intended to write a short paper, which you might incorporate with your report if you thought proper, but in the press of other duties I have been compelled to abandon it."

From Dr. Patterson I received an interesting communication upon the general causes affecting the mental health, more particularly of women in country districts, which will be found in another portion of the present memoir.

Willing as I should have been to have incorporated the opinions of my colleagues to a greater extent in this report, whether or no they were confirmatory of my own, it will be seen that I am compelled in great measure to assume its sole responsibility.

II. — Point previously attained.

Reference has been made in the letters of these gentlemen to views concerning the causation of insanity in women that I had already expressed. These will be found in full, or in abstract, in the published proceedings of the American Academy of Arts and Sciences for 1864-5, and in various numbers of the Boston Medical and Surgical Journal for the same period. It may be that the experience of others, if carefully analyzed, will not wholly confirm me in the position that I have assumed; the lapse of many months (now several years), however, since I first threw out a hint of my convictions, in the report of the Massachusetts State Commission on Insanity for 1863-4, has but served to render me the more decided in my every assumption, and I believe it will be found, just as it was with my statements concerning the frequency of criminal abortion, — a report upon which, as chairman of the special committee upon this subject, I had the honor to render to the American Medical Association in 1859,* — that though my premises

---

* To my colleagues upon that committee, Drs. Blatchford, of New York, Hodge, of Pennsylvania, Pope, of Missouri, Barton, of South Carolina, Lopez, of Alabama, Semmes, of the District of Columbia, and Brisbane, of Wisconsin, all of them gentlemen much older and of higher standing in the profession than myself (and three or four of whom have now deceased), I shall always feel under deep obligations for the brave and sympathetic alacrity with which they indorsed views that at the time seemed to many, of an earlier school, heretical or unfounded.

were so startling, and of so practical results as to be by many denied, more careful and more general investigation has shown that they were in reality very much understated.

Preliminarily, I wish it distinctly understood, —

1. That I assert for the insanity of women neither a universality of causation or of treatment. As I have already been misinterpreted upon both these points in my previous writings, clearly as I endeavored to express myself, the disclaimer now made is not unnecessary.

2. I have shown that in the writings of alienists, there is comparatively very little to be found in acknowledgment of the part played by her *sex* in the causation and prolongation of insanity in women. As regards suggestion, approbation, or demand of a consequent and rational treatment, even less than this can be produced from the authors referred to.

I do not state, however, that the key to insanity in women has not long been in possession of these gentlemen, but I prove by the facts adduced, that though they may have possessed it, they have not appreciated that the theory referred to would unlock, what has always been in every asylum, as in every psychological text-book, a sealed question and an opprobrium. They have not used it for this purpose in their annual reports, in their memoirs, in their published statistics, or in their medical treatment.

3. I have alleged that in a very large proportion of the cases of insanity occurring in woman, her sex is in reality the predisposing, the exciting, or the continuing cause of the malady; but I do not assert that there are never present other predisposing, exciting, or continuing causes at work efficiently in women as in men.

4. I have claimed that from the above premises it follows that the treatment of insane women should, in many instances, be of a direct and physical character; but this, it will be allowed, is a very different thing from teaching that the treatment of insane women should always and only be local; which I have never advised, and which I should myself be the first to condemn.

5. As a means, and only as a means, towards the end at which we all are aiming, namely, the cure of the patient, I have endeavored to exhibit the necessity at every asylum of a board of consulting physicians, skilled in the diagnosis and treatment of uterine disease, which is now acknowledged to especially require erudite tact and an appreciative mind; but I have distinctly stated that such aid was only to be made use of at the discretion of the superintendent, whose monarchical and exclusive sway, legislative and executive, economical and financial, spiritual and corporeal, could thus in no wise be lessened or interfered with.

If superintendents are not in reality afraid of a shadow, if they are not disinclined to allow the profession at large to participate in the study of mind diseased, why this tone of suspicion, or jealousy, or fear that a simple, needed, and practical suggestion by a medical man who knows whereof he is speaking, has in certain quarters called forth?

I have ventured to direct the attention of the profession to the results then and now again to be placed before them, as in every respect important, and in some respects novel. Their right to this last attribute has been challenged, and in a quarter where, in view of all the circumstances, we should have last looked for any counter claim. I refer to a statement by the editor-in-chief of the official organ of American Superintendents, Dr. John P. Gray, of the Utica Asylum.* Abundant evidence will be afforded in the present paper to settle all doubt upon this score.

I merely wish thus beforehand to define my position; asserting as new only the attempt to apply upon the large scale to the treatment of insane women, in asylums as in private practice, views that in theory were partially recognized even by Hippocrates, though they have been practically acted upon by few or none of his successors.

My position is rather that of the pioneer than of the discoverer. There is little positively new in

* MS. Letter of December, 1864.

medicine; there is much that is comparatively so. Not a statement, however original, to which a previous clew has not existed and cannot be found. Not a psychologist, however practically he may disbelieve in a local origin for mental derangement, and may have put his disbelief on permanent record, but might aver that such origin were perfectly familiar to him; that he learned it in his mother's womb, or imbibed it from her bosom, even that he inherited its knowledge from his ancestors, for cases enough were on record in their day and from time immemorial.

I have referred to a disposition on the part of certain individuals, apparently very few in number, to misinterpret or to undervalue facts that may be stated, or deductions that may be drawn, by any one who is not professedly a psychological specialist, and upon that ground. I shall therefore take the liberty of fortifying some of the points that I shall make, by the evidence or the language of gentlemen whose position within the inner circle alluded to is such as to render their authority unquestioned.

For instance — and as it is a question that met me upon the very threshold of this report, I have little hesitation in presenting it. What shall be allowed to render a man conversant with the various phases of mental disturbance? One superintendent, the physician to the Utica Asylum, considers that it can only be attained by prolonged residence in an insane hospital. Under date of January, 11th ult. (1865), he writes me as follows, and in expressing an opinion as to views of my own, unless it was arrived at very superficially or at second hand, he must have been aware that they were based upon no isolated case or two, but upon a dozen years of almost exclusive observation, upon the most extended scale, of sick women. He says, —

> "It certainly appears to me that some practical experience in the management and treatment of the insane, acquired not from an isolated case or two, but in some large hospital, would greatly modify your ideas. You would then have an opportunity of ascertaining what is really known on the subject, and what treatment is actually practised in these institutions."

On the other hand, it is possible that careful comparisons of the actual working detail of many hospitals, of the plans, medical and in other respects, under which they are conducted, and of the ideas of their respective superintendents as afforded by their various systems of treatment, seen in operation, and described personally by the gentlemen themselves, may perhaps give even a better knowledge of what is really known on the subject, and what treatment is actually practised in these institutions, than a residence, no matter for what length of time, at any asylum in the land. In no matter is the old saying of Morgagni more true than in this: *Perpendendæ, non numerandæ, sunt observationes.*

Is a knowledge of psychological literature sufficient to make one a safe guide? There is, I will venture to say, no department of medicine, save the closely-allied and more properly considered pseudo-science, phrenology, whose literature is so crowded with contradictory statements and conflicting theories, with utterly baseless generalizations and facts misinterpreted, as this department of insanity. Each successive text-book has repeated the errors, or many of them, of its predecessors. There are, it is true, notable exceptions, the various works of Ray, for instance — which are all of them, for originality of thought, for closeness of observation, and for justness of reasoning, veritable oases in this most barren of deserts; but even Bucknill and Tuke, whose book is in many respects one of the best of modern medicine, still retain the old, and that ought to be obsolete, artificial classification; which, last relic of an ancient nosology, would separate all the forms of insanity in accordance with their several symptoms, and by ignoring the great and fundamental question of their causation, would reduce to a matter of unsafe and blind routine their chance of cure. Each author, moreover, and often without a word of credit, repeats the details, insufficient or irrelevant though they may be, of cases that seem to have been handed down from time almost immemorial, judging from the distance backward to which in several instances I have traced them.

It was my first intention to have presented in this report a summary of all the cases on record, so far as I could collect them, illustrative of the diagnosis, positive and differential, that had been formed, and of the treatment of insanity in women by past and present masters in psychological medicine; and for this purpose I had tabulated or made minutes of a mass of cases, amounting probably to several hundreds; but, upon more carefully examining them, they were found so faulty, or so imperfectly reported, as for all practical purposes to be useless.

What, for instance, shall I say of the fact, that while in scores and in hundreds of cases great care has been taken to say whether the woman had or had not had the itch, — for this affection was formerly considered an important agent in the causation of insanity, — in scarcely any, on the other hand, however plainly connected with pelvic derangement, is any physical examination mentioned or its results given; a method of studying and reporting that does not seem to have ceased with the years bygone. Or, what of the similar fact that, in the autopsies of the insane, it has seldom seemed necessary to critically examine other organs of the body than the brain, even though that showed no trace whatever of lesion. Or what, again, of the other fact, still almost universal, that in the cases of undoubted pelvic origin or influence, — at least, in those that have been reported, — where attempts at physical exploration have been made, precise mention is omitted of the exact species of local disease that was ascertained to be present, so important in deciding as to whether the means resorted to for its relief were exactly what were required, without which correspondence it is evident a cure could not be hoped, and a failure to effect it could prove no error as to the ultimate causation of the mental disturbance. A mind that has been trained in the arena of modern general practice, and is accustomed to depend only upon the most rigid and rigorous methods of diagnosis, finds little in such faulty material that either satisfies or is edifying.

Let me give, upon this point, a single forcible word from one of the best psychological authorities in this country, Dr. Workman, of Toronto, the superintendent of the immense government asylum of Canada West. He writes me as follows: —

"So much has been written on insanity, as I am sure you know, the tendency of which has only been to becloud the subject, that even when one is fortunate enough to command a good proportion of the works, he has to wade through terrible cesspool accumulations, or scramble over piles of forsaken habitations, before he dare venture to say to the world that he has begun to study."

With this word of explanation, which will have been seen to be necessary, I proceed.

III. — Work to be done.

I had intended to have presented in this report a carefully prepared and somewhat complete essay upon the insanity of women, it being my opinion, as stated in my paper published in the volume of the Transactions of the Association for 1865, —

I. That in women mental disease is often, perhaps generally, dependent upon functional or organic disturbance of the reproductive system.

II. That in women the access or exacerbation of mental disease is usually coincident with the catamenial establishment, its periodical access, temporary suppression, or final cessation. And, therefore, —

III. That the rational and successful treatment of mental disease in women must be based upon the preceding theories, which I have claimed are established, —

1. By many analogies, physiological and pathological, in the cerebral manifestations of the human female and that of the lower mammals.

2. By clinical observation; and, —

3. By the results of autopsies of the insane, both in private practice and, where made with equal care and impartiality, in insane asylums.

To cover, however, properly all the ground that I had marked out would occupy a larger space than, perhaps, one has a right to claim for a single report; and since it was commenced, I have received communications, published and private, of such a character as have satisfied me that it is better at this time and in this place to strike boldly at the very root of the present system of theory and management of insanity in women, before attempting to train a healthier and sturdier growth in its stead. Convinced of being correct in this, I intend, health permitting, to pursue it; and, to prove that I am in earnest, now subjoin a sketch of the essay that I have already partially prepared for submitting to the Association.

I. Causation.

The insanity of woman proved generally **peripheral and reflex** —
  1. By evidence negative.
     a. Admissions of psychologists.
        α. Cerebral disease without **insanity**.
        β. Insanity without cerebral disease.
     b. Omission of autopsies.
     c. Neglect at autopsies.
     d. Results of autopsies.
        α. At asylums.
        β. At general hospitals.
        γ. In civil practice.
  2. By evidence positive.
     a. Analogies from —
        α. Other sympathetic results.
           I. On nerves sensory.
           II. On nerves motor.
           III. On functions **organic.**
         * IV. On functions animal.
           V. On fœtus in utero.
        β. Madness in lower mammals.

γ. Admissions —
  I. Of psychologists.
  II. Of gynæcologists.
  III. Of women themselves.
δ. Cases on record.
  I. Psychical.
  II. Obstetrical.
ε. Cases now first given.
ζ. Autopsies —
  I. On record.
  II. Now first given.
η. Time of development.
  I. Fœtal.
  II. Congenital.
  III. Puberal.
  IV. Catamenial.
  V. Nuptal.
  VI. Gestal.
  VII. Puerperal.
  VIII. Lacteal.
  IX. Climaxal.
  X. Senile.
  XI. Organic disease.
θ. Effect of treatment —
  I. At asylums.
  II. In civil practice.
ι. Reflex induction of cerebral derangement.
κ. Reflex cure of cerebral derangement.
λ. Not necessary to expect uterine disease always to produce insanity, even if it were allowed that insanity in women were usually induced by uterine disease.

II. Theory of ultimate causation.
  1. Effect on general health —
    a. Of pain.
    b. Of abnormal flux.
      α. Hemorrhagic.
      β. Leucorrhœal.
      γ. Lacteal.

2. Cerebral irritation.
    a. Direct.
    b. Reflex.
3. Circulation of carbon, uneliminated
    a. By lungs.
    b. By uterus.
        α. In virginity.
        β. In pregnancy.
            I. Healthy.
            II. Diseased.
4. Dystocia.
5. Uterine inheritance.
    α. Metritic.
    β. Placental.
6. Toxæmia.
III. Indications of Prevention.
IV. Indications of Rational Treatment.
    1. To ascertain the primary lesion.
    2. To prevent exacerbating influences.
    3. To relieve physical symptoms.
    4. To remove the exciting cause, it being of no slight moment —
        a. At what stage a patient is treated.
        b. And in what way she is treated, whether
            α. According to the individual case, or
            β. By routine.

It will be perceived that there is much that can be said that I believe has not been said upon this most interesting and practical topic, just as there is much that can be done that has not yet been done towards relieving or curing its unfortunate victims. I have now at hand a large mass of material, original and collected, concerning the various points above indicated, that I shall hope to present to the profession at some future period.

In the mean time I shall endeavor to take by the horns one or two little chimeras that have been shaken at me, or at any rate to look them in the face.

It has been asserted, in communications addressed to me since I have been appointed upon this committee, or in publications intended to break down, to discredit, or to ridicule my testimony, —

1. That insanity in women is seldom dependent upon a pelvic cause.

2. That it has so frequently been recognized as thus dependent, that any discussion of the subject is unnecessary.

3. That thorough physical examinations of insane women are already generally made whenever required.

4. That such are not required.

5. That they would be positively injurious to the patient herself, and, if in an asylum, to the other patients, and to general discipline.

It will be hardly possible for me to give to each of these contradictory points the attention their importance deserves, although I am prepared, in each instance, to show their utter worthlessness.

In what, however, I shall say, I shall endeavor, so far as possible, to take my arguments from psychologists themselves, using, in the main, their own words, originally written though these may have been for a different purpose, and in ignorance of the real character and meaning of the facts described. Were these gentlemen aware of the inconsistencies, both in theory and practice, that are everywhere recorded in their special literature, they would be much more careful than one or two of them have lately been; for it is evident, —

1. That if my views are true, but yet long known, then local examination and treatment ought not to have been stated to be generally unnecessary or positively injurious; and, —

2. That, if they are false, then it cannot be claimed that they have long been recognized as well founded, and, in practice, daily carried out to the letter, both of which conflicting assertions have been made by gentlemen claiming to be leaders in the specialty of insanity.

Due allowances are, of course, to be made for a certain measure of professional conservatism, however arrogantly expressed; and I do not entirely indorse, though I quote, the following remarks by Dr. Galt, of Virginia, himself a superintendent, and then of the Eastern Asylum. They are none the less pertinent, however, as coming from that source, and as made to rebuke the tendency of an older school to repress innovation, or even inquiry.

"The laudator temporis acti is so common, that we do not think it necessary to quote the opinions of the past on the present subject. As a general rule, writers allow a change to be effected, if, as they say, it is feasible. But such a mode of argument is no longer admissible. He who opposes the proposed arrangement, must be prepared to defend himself on the assertion of its intrinsic inferiority. Admitting, however, such fancies to stand for what they are worth, we still find the medical world divided as to the matter in question; and this circumstance itself should induce us to lean to the new views, because every one is aware of the prejudices which association weaves about established customs and regulations. It is said that when Harvey declared to the world his discovery of the circulation of the blood, no physician beyond forty years of age gave in his adhesion to the new views." *

IV. — THE BRAIN THE SEAT OF INSANITY, NOT ALWAYS OF ITS CAUSE.

I have dared to say, that, in my opinion, the ancient and still usual classification of insanity, which artificially divides the forms of mental aberration according to their mental peculiarities, is faulty and erroneous. Such a method of classifying disease according to its symptoms alone, would not, at the present day, be tolerated in any other department of medicine. It is the more necessary to dwell for a few moments upon the question here involved, for it lies at the foundation of this report; and upon its decision depends, in great measure, the truth of my views concerning the insanity of women, novel or trite as these may prove.

Dr. Workman, of Toronto, to whom I have already alluded, seems to have argued more boldly and more

---

* American Journal of Insanity, xi. 229.

ably for the extra-cerebral causation of insanity than, perhaps, any other writer in this country, both in his own writings and his late translation of Schrœder van der Kolk's little work upon the pathology and theraupeutics of insanity, in the American Superintendents' Journal.* He writes me as follows: —

"What can be more exact, what more rational, what more practically suitable than the assignment of all cases of insanity to the two grand heads, idiopathic and sympathetic? in other words, fixing all insanity either *in* the brain or *out* of it. It has long been my belief that, unless in confirmed low dementia and idiocy, insanity has no *necessary* connection with *diseased* brain, properly so called. I believe that when appreciable, palpable disease exists in the brain, we always have something *besides*, and something *essentially* different from insanity. It does not satisfy me to be told that disease in the brain may exist and be undetectable. We do not admit this assertion in application to any other organ or structure. If you ask me to admit the presence of disease in the eye, or the ear, or the lungs, and fail, by scalpel or microscope to demonstrate it, am I sceptic because I refuse credence?

"The circular argument of starting with the premises, that, as the brain is the organ of the mind, and insanity is a disease of the mind, therefore the brain, in insanity, must be diseased, whether we detect the disease or not, has, it appears to me, been too long deferred to. The fallacy here may exist in any one, or in all, the terms of the syllogism.

"1. I would say I do not comprehend the term 'organ of the mind.' I understand the terms organ of sight, organ of taste, organ of digestion, of circulation, of urination, &c., &c.; but where is the parallelism, or even the resemblance, between these functions and thought?

"2. What is meant by *disease* of mind? What is the

---

* American Journal of Insanity, April and July, 1864, p. 63, &c.

parallelism, or even remote resemblance, between any form of bodily disease and mental abnormality?

"3. Why should a diseased brain be essential to insanity? If it is absent in a single case, its presence cannot be essential. I believe it is absent in *many* cases, yea, in the majority of cases. Have you carefully noted the mental condition of persons dying under pulmonary consumption? and, if so, have you not often been struck with its close approximation to insanity? Pulmonary disease is present in a very large proportion of cases of insanity, and I believe in incurable cases it is present in fully one half. We may, or we may not, discover cerebral lesion *super*-added — very generally I think *not*. This fact is surely one of much significance.

"In *all* emotional insanity of women, and especially in the religious forms, I am persuaded the generative organs play a most important part. I would almost say, they give the ground-tone."

I shall now proceed to show, —

1. That while the brain is undoubtedly the seat of insanity, yet it is not necessarily the seat of its cause.

2. And that this is proved by *à priori* reasoning, and, both negatively and positively, by the results of autopsies.

3. That while idiopathic insanity, requiring direct cerebral or simply moral treatment alone, is very rare, sympathetic or reflex insanity, requiring treatment of a special character, is extremely common.

4. And that, on the one hand, such reflex causation is and should be much more common in females than in males, while, on the other hand, of the various forms of it occurring in females, the majority of them are owing to functional or organic diseases of the

uterus and its appendages; in other words, that they are of a sexual character.

These facts I shall support at this time only by the evidence of superintendents themselves, by no means exhausting the testimony of this character that I have at hand, nor drawing upon the extensive material that is afforded me from other quarters, which I shall reserve for a future communication upon the subject, that may hereafter be made by me to the profession.

The first witness whom I call is Dr. Ray, of the Butler Hospital, at Providence, R. I. (now, 1870, of Philadelphia).

"It can hardly be necessary, at the present time," says this gentleman, "to prove the fact of the dependence of the mind on the brain for its external manifestations; that, in short, the brain is the material organ of the intellectual and effective powers. Whatever opinion may be entertained of the nature of the mind, it is generally admitted, at least by all enlightened physiologists, that it must of necessity be put in connection with matter, and that the brain is the part of the body by means of which this connection is effected. Little as we know beyond this single fact, it is enough to warrant the inference that derangement of the structure, or of the vital actions, of the brain, must be followed by abnormal manifestations of the mind, and, consequently, that the presence of the effect indicates the existence of the cause. Whether the morbid action arises in the digestive or some other system, and is reflected thence to the brain by means of the nervous sympathies, or arises primarily in the brain, the soundness of the above principle is equally untouched. This leads us to the source of the hesitation that has been evinced by pathologists to consider the brain as the seat of insanity.

"From the fact that organic lesions are not always discoverable after death in the brains of the subjects of insanity, it has been inferred that the brain is not the seat of this disease; though, if this fact were true, — it being also true that no other organ in the body invariably presents marks of organic derangement in insanity, — the only legitimate inference would have been, that, in some cases, it is impossible to discover such lesions by any means in our power. The strangest theoretical error which this soundness of the brain in some cases has occasioned, is that of denying the existence of any material affection at all, and attributing the disease entirely to an affection of the immaterial principle. If the same pathological principles had guided men's reasoning, respecting this disease, that they have applied to the investigation of others, this error would never have been committed. It will scarcely be contended, at the present day, at least, that the structural changes found after death, from any disease, are the primary cause of the disturbances manifested by symptoms during life, or that, if the interior could be inspected at the beginning of the disease, any of these structural changes would be discovered. It is now a well-recognized principle that such changes must be preceded by some change in the vital actions of the part where they occur. This vital change is now generally expressed by the term *irritation*, and nothing is implied by it relative to the nature of this change more than an exaltation of action. Irritation, then, is the initial stage of disease — the first in the chain of events, of which disorganization is the last; and, of course, nothing can be more unphilosophical than to attribute disturbances of function exclusively to any structural changes that may take place during the progress of these successive stages." *

To what pathological actions or structural changes is the brain then liable? And here I present the evidence of Dr. Bucknill, of England, medical super-

* Medical Jurisprudence of Insanity, pp. 128-130.

intendent of the Devon County Lunatic Asylum. He tells us, —

"As an organ abundantly supplied with blood vessels, the brain is obviously liable to all abnormal conditions, which irregularities in the quality or quantity of the blood, and the relation thereof to its tissue, can occasion; it is liable to anæmia and to hyperæmia, both passive and active, and to the latter accompanied by organizable and unorganizable exudates. It is also more readily acted upon by various chemical changes in the blood than any other organ. Excess of carbon or defect of oxygen tells first upon it; and many substances in the blood which affect other organs little, or not at all, affect this noblest of the organs with intense force. All diseases, therefore, which depend upon the movement or quantity of the blood, and many of those which depend upon its quality, are the fruitful source of abnormal cerebral conditions. There are, it is true, many blood-poisons and diseases which do not affect the brain. Thus, it is strange, that although the gout-poison affects the temper strongly, and often endangers the intellect, that of rheumatism has no effect thereon. Tuberculosis, moreover, while attacking every other organ of the body, very rarely affects the adult cerebrum. But the brain is liable to a species of disturbance, apparently quite unconnected with the quality, quantity, or movement of the blood, a species of disturbance to which other organs are liable only in a modified and unimportant degree. We allude to the disturbance caused by sympathy with injuries of, or noxious influences applied to, peripheral portions of the nervous system.*

These sympathetic disturbances, however, occasioned by the irritation of some part of the distal nervous system, do not necessarily produce any anatomical changes, if the examination is made during

* Manual of Psychological Medicine, p. 349.

the early period of the disease.* After a while, the brain may pass from the state of physiological excitement into that of pathological change, and alterations in its structure then be found on examination, although this is by no means necessarily the case.

"The condition of the cerebral substance is the prime question in the pathology of mental disease. Frequently this condition can only be judged of by the state of its blood vessels, or can only be guessed at by that of its membranes, or some still more remote indication. Not unfrequently, in partial and sympathetic insanity, it appears to be perfectly sound in structure, although the deductions of science assure us that this soundness is in appearance only, and is solely attributable to the imperfection of our means of observing and investigating.

"To the pathologist the substance of the brain is as yet practically structureless. Although the microscope reveals cells and tubes, and intervening stroma, up to the present time it is unable to indicate when they are in a normal or abnormal state; and although it may prove that in some cases the smaller arteries are diseased, that in a few others there are exudation-corpuscles, or an increase of fatty particles in the substance itself, it has not yet enabled us to distinguish between the states of the whole organ, which must be diametrically opposite — for instance, between the state of hypertrophy and atrophy." †

Let us again listen to Dr. Ray.

"It has been stated by Foderè, in explanation of the pathological causes that produce the alternation of paroxysms and lucid intervals so constantly seen in certain forms of insanity, that the former are attended by an excessive plethora of the blood vessels of the brain, and the latter by a relaxed, atonic condition of these vessels, which is an effect

---

* Manual of Psychological Medicine, p. 403.
† Ibid., p. 421.

of their previous forcible distention. In this condition they are liable to be suddenly engorged by exciting causes, such as intemperance in eating or drinking, anger, violent exercise, insolation, &c.; or in consequence of a certain predisposition of constitution. It is, indeed, well known that the return of the paroxysms is often retarded by regulated diet, bleeding, quiet, seclusion, kind treatment, and the absence of the above named stimuli. It is thus shown conclusively that in every lucid interval there remains some unsoundness of the material organ of the mind, which may be designated generally as a morbid irritability, which, on the application of the slightest exciting cause, may produce an outbreak of mania in all its original severity." *

"But," asks Andral, in his Clinique Médicale, "when we have referred the symptoms to hyperæmia in one case, and to anæmia in another, are we to come to the bottom of the subject? By no means," he replies to his own question; for this hyperæmia and this anæmia are themselves mere effects, which — a thing very remarkable — the same influence can very often produce.

In Esquirol's great work upon maladies of the mind, published so recently as 1838, his opinions on pathology, which had been in accordance with those still so generally held concerning the insane, will be found to have been considerably modified. Referring to the case of a recent maniac, who was killed by one of her companions, and in whose body he and his pupils were surprised to find no lesions of the brain or its meninges, he declares that pathological anato-

---

* Medical Jurisprudence of Insanity, p. 339.

my, in spite of the very important labors of Foville, Calmeil, Bayle, Guislain, and others, has not been able to make us acquainted with the organic cause of mania. He says, —

"Thirty years ago I would willingly have written upon the pathological cause of madness. At the present day I would not attempt a labor so difficult, so much of incertitude and contradiction is there in the results of the necroscopy of the insane made up to this time. But I may add that modern researches permit us to hope for ideas more positive, more clear, and more satisfactory."

We are now naturally conducted to the actual results of post-mortem examinations of the insane. I again quote Esquirol: —

"From this announcement, every one might expect that we should be able to point out the seat of insanity, and to make known the nature and seat of the organic lesion, of which insanity is the expression. This we can by no means accomplish. The examinations of the dead have, to the present period, been barren of practical information. The facts observed by Willis, Manget, Bonnet, Morgagni, Gunz, Meckel, Greding, Vicq d'Azyr, Camper, Chaussier, Gall, and others, have produced only negative or contradictory results.

"All the labor that has been expended upon the anatomy of the brain has produced no other result than a more exact description of this organ, and the despairing certainty of our being forever unable to assign to its parts the uses from whence we may derive information with reference to the exercise of the thinking faculty, whether in health or disease.

"Before drawing any conclusions," continues this great authority, "from these organic lesions observed among the insane, will it not be well to acquaint ourselves with all the varieties, both of the cranium and of the brain, which are compatible with the integrity of the faculties of the understanding? Would not this be the true point of departure for all our pathological researches? Now, says the learned Chaussier, there is no organ in which we find greater varieties, with respect to volume, weight, density, and its respective proportions, than the brain. Have we carefully distinguished the results of concomitant maladies, or those diseases which terminate the life of the insane, from those which belong to mental alienation?

"Organic lesions of the brain reveal themselves by other signs than insanity. Thus, chronic inflammation of the meninges produces compression, which reveals itself by paralysis; cerebral hemorrhage is also manifested by paralysis. Tubercle, cancer, and softening of the brain present peculiar characters, which cannot be confounded with mental alienation. Have we reflected on the sudden and instantaneous cures of insanity? It is in consequence of having neglected these considerations that we reason so erroneously respecting the seat of this malady."*

Let us see what light upon these points has been afforded by actual study of the dead.

Autopsies are comparatively seldom made of the insane who die at asylums. The reason, or one reason, of this will have been already made evident — examination of the brain, so barren of result, having usually alone been made. Upon this point I will reproduce evidence that I have already elsewhere presented.†

"Many who have professed familiarity with these subjects have asserted that the morbid appearances found in the bodies of the insane were unworthy of record; they should rather have confessed that they were unable to

---

* Mental Maladies, p. 69.
† Boston Med. and Surg. Journal, April, 1864, p. 198.

appreciate their value. With the more thorough and complete investigation of these matters, we may hope eventually to arrive at some correct views as to the nature of those laws, the transgression of which leads to sensorial disturbance, but no approach to the truth can be made except through the portal of morbid anatomy, which has revealed this important fact, that the record of post-mortem examinations, as preserved in an asylum for the insane, differs in most striking and essential particulars from that preserved in a general public hospital." *

"Autopsies," said Dr. Douglass to me, when visiting the Government Asylum of Lower Canada at Beaufort, near Quebec, then under his charge, "autopsies of the insane no one ever thinks of making in Canada, save that enthusiast whom you have been visiting at Toronto." While, on the other hand, it is from this very enthusiast at Toronto, Dr. Workman, to whom I have already alluded, that the profession is indebted for some of the most important of the steps towards elucidating the real pathology and ultimate causation of insanity in its reflex manifestations, that have ever yet been made.

Dr. Hunt, formerly of the Hartford Asylum, has put the following admission on record: —

"The number of post-mortem examinations made in the hospitals for the treatment of insanity in this country is very few, and of this number fewer still are ever published. The cause is evident, and is not likely very soon to be obviated." †

---

* Holmes Coote: Journal of Psychological Medicine, vol. iv. p. 384.

† I freely acknowledge that in some instances, as was stated by Drs Choate and Bemis at the meeting of Superintendents held at Providence (Am. Jour. of Insanity, July, 1862), it is difficult or impossible to obtain the consent of

The examination, which was permitted me, of the very extended, minute, and most suggestive pathological records at Toronto, furnished proof that this paucity of autopsies is owing neither to " want of opportunity,"* nor to dearth of practical results, when properly looked for.

It is proved, however, from abundant evidence, that,

1. Insanity may exist without structural changes of the brain, and that,

2. Structural changes of the brain may exist without insanity.

"It must be admitted," says Dr. Bucknill, "that we are not yet in a position, as regards our knowledge of the morbid appearances of the brain, to base our nosology upon the revelations of the dead-houses. We can only wait an advance of knowledge which will render this possible." †

The late Dr. Bell, of the McLean Asylum, at Somerville, justly considered one of our most reliable authorities, has left no doubtful expression of his own opinion, which was, that autopsies of the insane generally present no material lesion of the brain; changes, indeed, there are to be seen, but only those that may have occurred in articulo mortis.‡

---

a patient's friends to have a post-mortem examination; but this difficulty obtains to nearly an equal degree at general hospitals, where, nevertheless, such examinations are much more common.

* Translation of Esquirol, p. 233.
† Loc. citat., p. 94.
‡ American Journal of Insanity, x. p. 79.

Upon another occasion he stated that my friend, the late Dr. Waldo I. Burnett, of Boston, one of the most accomplished microscopists in the country, had made examinations of the brain of persons who had died in a state of chronic insanity, but had been unable to discover any change of structure whatever, or any sign to indicate that it did not belong to an individual whose mind was unaffected.*

Dr. Bucknill observes, —

"The brains of the insane appear to be certainly not more liable than those of others to various incidental affections. Thus, in four hundred autopsies of the insane, we have only once met with a hydatid, only once with tubercular deposit in the substance and meninges, only once with a fibro-cellular tumor, and not once with malignant disease. The arteries at the base do not appear to be more frequently or extensively affected with atheromatous change than those of sane persons of the same age; and in the bodies of the insane we have never yet met with that cretaceous deposit in the coats of the small arteries, which makes them feel like pieces of fine wire imbedded in the brain-substance. We have never met with that leather-like and fibro-cartilaginous hardness or resistance to which sclerosis of the brain is described to attain. The two forms of ramollissement are not found more frequently in the brains of persons dying insane than in those of others. The same may be said of the cellular infiltration described by Durand Fardel, with which in four hundred autopsies we have met but twice.

"A large number of brains of the insane we have diligently investigated with a first-rate microscope. The results appear to us to have afforded no distinction between the sane and the insane brain. We have found exudation corpuscles, but only in instances where the existence of inflammatory

---

* American Journal of Insanity, xi. 1854, p. 53.

action was apparent without the use of the microscope; and, therefore, this microscopic test of cerebral inflammation, proposed by Dr. Hughes Bennett, appears to be of little value. In inflammatory and softened parts of the brain-substance we have found fatty degeneration of the coats of the small arteries; but it remains to be seen whether this change is not as frequent in the brains of the sane. We have not been able to discover fatty degeneration of the arteries where the pathological changes more peculiar to insanity alone existed. The same may be said of fatty degeneration of the brain-substance, consisting in the abundant dissemination of amorphous fat particles, which is found in some specimens of cerebral softening.

"It seemed reasonable to expect that, by the aid of the microscope, one would be able to ascertain whether any exudation or addition to the stroma of the brain, or any change in size, shape, or proportionate number of its cells, takes place; and in the indurated brain of chronic insanity, whether that finely fibrillated exudate, which has been described by some writers, actually exists; also, whether, in extreme atrophy of the brain, any proportion exists in the diminution or degeneration in the form of the cells or tubes. In none of these points of inquiry have we been able to attain the slightest success." *

It could hardly be expected, when the contents of the cranial cavity throw so little light upon the pathological character of insanity, that a study of its exterior could be productive of fruitful results. Such, however, has been assiduously attempted, but the results are neither uniform nor undoubted.

"Although we believe" — it is Bucknill who is now speaking — "that the average dimensions of the head are below those of the sane, when the comparison is obtained by the examination of large numbers, still, in a great number of

* Loc. citat., p. 430.

instances, they will be found to be good: and, indeed, the head is frequently not only large, but phrenologically well-shaped.

"We are not aware in what proportion of the sane the shape of the head is peculiar, since it is rare that opportunities occur for making the observation among them; but among the insane a considerable proportion present decided peculiarities in the shape of the cranium. The most frequent one is a want of symmetry in the two sides. One side is rather flatter or smaller than the other, or the whole cranium is pushed over a little to one side, or one side is a little more forward than the other, or the two anomalies coexist, giving the cranium a sort of twisted appearance. These things will not be seen unless they are looked for, with accurate and careful eyes, upon the shaven scalp.

"Sometimes the skull is high and domelike; more frequently it is as if it had been compressed laterally, and elongated from before backwards — heel-shaped, in fact, like the skulls figured by Dr. Minchin,* in which the centres of ossification of the parietal bones are increased in number. Sometimes the forehead is preternaturally flat, narrow, or receding, or very large and bulging, or the occipital region is deficient, and the back of the head rises in a straight line with the nape of the neck. Sometimes the skull has a remarkably square configuration. The square and carinated form of skull we have most frequently seen in connection with mania; the domelike and high, vertical skull, and also the unsymmetrical skull, most frequently in melancholia. In mania the anterior cranium is more frequently of good shape and size than in melancholia. In the latter the forehead is often small and mean, but sometimes it is disproportionately large and globose. The shape of the head, indicated by the rules of phrenologists, can only fairly be expected to coincide with the mental symptoms in those somewhat rare instances in which insanity is the mere development in excess of natural character; and in some such instances we have found the shape of the head

* Dublin Medical Journal.

tally, in its general outline, with the indications of phrenology.

"Occasionally depressions are found in the outer skull, which sometimes do, and sometimes do not, correspond with the bulging of the inner table of the cranium. When they do not correspond, we have found that they indicate a local absorbtion of the diploe.

"It is an interesting question how far the shape of the skull alters in insanity. If the forehead expands, even in mature age, under the influence of intellectual development, it is likely that it will contract under the influence of intellectual decay. Some writers have asserted that the shrinking of the brain in atrophy is commonly, and to a considerable extent followed, and the cranium filled, by a flattening and shrinking of the cranial bones.* Rokitansky also affirms that atrophy of the brain frequently gives rise to deposit of bone on the inner table of the skull, especially about the anterior convolutions.

"We have not satisfied ourselves that the increased thickness of the cranium, which is frequently met with in the insane, is in any way connected with atrophy of the brain. Some of the thickest and heaviest craniums which we have met with have occurred in instances in which there was little or no cerebral atrophy; and the condition of the cranium, where there is undoubted atrophy of the brain, is not unfrequently one of abnormal tenuity." †

Thus it is seen not merely that there is no direct correspondence between the exterior of the skull and mental integrity, any more than between the exterior of the skull and the shape and consistence of its contents. We constantly see all the degrees of irregularity and excess or deficiency of cranial development that have been described, in every-day life, and coin-

* Paget: Lectures on Pathology.
† Loc. citat., p. 410.

cident with perfect sanity. while even in idiocy it is not necessary that the normal symmetry shall at all be lacking, though this is undoubtedly frequently the case.

It must not be concluded, from the examples of microcephalous idiots, that a small head is a necessary accompaniment of idiocy. "On the contrary," says Dr. Tuke, Medical Officer to the York Retreat, "many idiots have large heads, leaving out of the question instances of hydrocephalus." Parchappe has stated, as the result of very careful inquiry, that if there exist a general relation between the volume of the brain and the degree of intelligence, "facts are wanting to deduce rigorously, from this relation, the different degrees of intellectual and moral capacity." Of one hundred idiotic heads examined by Belhomme, eighty-four presented more or less decided malformations of the forehead, occiput, and lateral portions. Twenty-five per cent. had a well-marked want of symmetry. On bringing together a hundred well-proportioned heads, he did not find a single idiot among the number. Gallice, after making a large number of observations, came to the conclusion, that the more intelligent the idiot is, the larger will be his head; but that this results from a greater development of the occiput. And this certainly accords with what Leuret had previously recorded, that the occiput in idiots is remarkably small.

Desmaisons, in his Memoir on the Form of the Head in Idiots, concludes that idiocy sometimes exists without any malformation; that it is impossible to fix upon any malformation peculiar to idiocy, when the volume of the head and its symmetry are retained; and that, in cases of this kind, flattening of the posterior portion of the head is as common as that of the forehead.* Gall laid it down as an axiom, that idiocy must exist when the head is not more than thirteen inches in circumference; and he says that the measurement of heads, in cases of complete imbecility, up to the ordinary exercise of the intellectual faculties, is comprehended between the following limits: The circumference varies from fourteen to seventeen inches, and the arc, between the root of the nose and the occipital foramen, measures nearly twelve. These dimensions, he adds, are accompanied with a greater or less degree of stupidity or fatuity, inability (more or less complete) of fixing the attention on a determinate object, vague sentiments, an irregular train of ideas, speech consisting of broken phrases, &c., and blind and irregular instincts.†

Esquirol's statements appear to be somewhat contradictory; for while a table of measurements, which he gives, exhibits a decided decrease in the size of the heads of idiots, he says, " The dimensions of the

---

* Manual of Psychological Medicine, p. 108.
† The Functions of the Brain, ii. p. 214.

crania of idiots are equal to those of other men," and concludes by exclaiming, " How much work there remains to accomplish, how much research, before we can state the coincidence of the volume and form of the head with the intellectual capacity!"

From the author last quoted I present the following conclusions: —

1. Vices of conformation in the cranium are met with only, or chiefly, among imbeciles, idiots, and cretins.

2. Organic lesions of the encephalon and its envelopes have been observed only among those whose insanity was complicated with paralysis, convulsions, and epilepsy, or rather these lesions appertain to the malady which has caused the death of the patients.

3. The sanguineous or serous effusions, the injections or infiltrations, which we meet with in the cranial cavity, the thickening of the meninges, their adhesions among themselves, with the cranium and the gray substance, the partial or general softening of the brain, the density of this organ, the fibrous, knotty, and cancerous tumors observed within the cranium, — all these alterations indicate either the causes or effects of insanity, or rather the effects of a complication to which the patients have yielded.

4. The alterations within the thorax, abdomen, and pelvic cavity are evidently independent of insanity. These alterations may, nevertheless, indicate the

source of mental alienation, by showing the organ primitively affected, which has reacted upon the brain.

5. All the organic lesions observed among the insane are found to exist among those who have never suffered from chronic delirium.

6. Many post-mortem examinations of the insane have revealed no alteration, although the insanity may have persisted for a great number of years.

7. Pathological anatomy shows us every part of the encephalon altered, in a state of suppuration, and destroyed, without chronic lesion of the understanding.

8. From the above data we may conclude that there are cases of insanity whose immediate cause escapes our means of investigation; that insanity depends upon an unknown modification of the brain; that it has not always its point of departure in the brain, but rather in the foci of sensibility, situated in different regions of the body, as disorders of the circulation do not always depend upon lesions of the heart, but upon those of some other portion of the vascular system.*

Lélut, who has also closely investigated this subject, sums up the result of his researches in the following words:—

"1. Numerous alterations of the brain and its envelopes are met with in delirium and insanity, especially in extreme

* Mental Maladies, p. 70.

forms of the latter; but these alterations are neither constant nor exclusive.

"2. Hence it must be allowed that the more or less local and coarse alterations in the skull, the brain, and its membranes, cannot be held to be the proximate causes of insanity. They are, doubtless, capable of existing with a delirious or insane condition; but they do not constitute this condition, and frequently they are only the exaggeration, the effect, or the transformation of it.

"3. That which may be given as the nearest approach to the proximate cause of delirium, and to the most acute form of insanity, is inflammatory lesion of the brain and its tunics. But this alteration neither does nor can constitute the state which is anterior to it, and may even destroy life without producing it.

"4. The conditions of the brain which approach the most closely to the proximate cause of the chronic forms of mental alienation, with or without impairment of motion, are without doubt chronic inflammation of the substance and of the membranes of the brain, its atrophy and induration, which may be accompanied by variations in its specific gravity. But yet these alterations are not the proximate cause of these forms of insanity, because they are neither constant nor exclusive, and they do not make themselves apparent except in an advanced period of the disease."*

These generalizations are carried to a still further extent by another writer upon the subject (Leuret), who states, —

1. That the authors who believe it possible to establish an anatomical change as the cause of insanity differ greatly among themselves. Thus Greding asserted that thickness of the bones of the cranium occurs in seventy-seven out of one hundred patients,

---

* Essay on the Value of Cerebral Alterations in Acute Delirium and Insanity.

while Haslam found this condition in ten only out of one hundred patients. Hyperæmia of the brain is recorded by Parchappe in forty-three cases out of one hundred, and by Bertoleni only in fourteen out of one hundred.

2. That some of the cerebral alterations to which insanity is attributed are by no means well established. Thus, in the cases which are cited of hypertrophy of the brain, it ought to have been shown that this was not owing to fulness of its vessels, or to the presence of a serosity in its tissue. These observations have not been made. Again, that which is called dense brain, or a soft brain, expresses nothing distinctly, except in extreme cases.

3. That the value attributed to certain alterations is deduced from a number of observations by far too small, so that one result frequently invalidates another. Thus Parchappe has deduced the average normal weight of the healthy brain from thirteen observations upon men, and nine upon women, and on this average he establishes the rule for atrophy of the brain. This average is evidently too small, and, indeed, Parchappe himself gives different averages elsewhere.

4. That the pathological alterations referred to insanity are met with in patients who have never been insane.

5. That all authors confess that there are insane

persons in whose brains no pathological changes are found.

6. That the lesions which are frequently met with among the insane, to which any value can be attached, are only met with in cases in which insanity has been complicated with paralysis; and that, in order to decide if any lesion is the cause of insanity, it is at least necessary to find it in a case of simple mental aberration, in which there has been no affection of motion or sensibility.*

The only answer that has been made, or that can be made, to these arguments, namely, that more minute methods of examination may perhaps be discovered which may show what the most powerful microscope as yet does not, is very unsatisfactory; the more so in view of the fact that the supposition of reflex causation is sufficient to account for every mystery, as it is allowed to do in neuralgia, tetanus, chorea, and hysteria. Dr. Bucknill is here at fault, and, like every other writer who falls back upon the brain as the seat of causation in insanity, proves inconsistent with himself.† It is possible that Brown-Séquard and John Dean, of Boston, may yet localize more disturbance in the brain, as they have so much in the spinal cord; but they cannot all.

What conclusion, then, with Esquirol, shall we

---

* The Moral Treatment of Insanity.
† Loc. cit., pp. 398-400.

draw from the facts that have now been presented? That the changes observed in the brain and its membranes are found in subjects who have given no indication of delirium; that organic lesions of the encephalon appertain to paralysis and convulsions rather than to dementia; and that the character and intensity of the delirium are not in proportion to the extent of the organic lesion. What shall we conclude? That the examinations of the bodies of the dead, which have so often furnished important information respecting the seat of disease, present no result which is satisfactory respecting the source and immediate cause of insanity. If in dementia there are indications of compression, sinking and collapse of the encephalon, is this state caused by the engorgement of the vascular system, or by the lessening of the cerebral circulation? Do not the arteries, having lost their elasticity or being ossified, propel with sufficient energy the blood which flows languidly in veins already too greatly dilated? Does not the inflammation of the meninges, by thickening the membranes, or by provoking a too abundant serous exhalation, induce the compression? Does not the contracting of the cranial cavity, by the separation of the internal table, particularly of the cranial portion, contribute to compress the brain? Post-mortem examinations teach us little in this respect; all the organic alterations of the brain or its dependencies appertaining less to the delirium than to its complications.*

Dr. Nichols, of Washington, Superintendent of the Government Hospital for the Insane, has expressed his opinion upon this subject in no uncertain language, " believing it highly important both to science and humanity. Therapeutists and pathologists," we are told, " are approaching, from different starting-points, a like rational, and what is much the most important, the *true* theoy of the proximate cause of insanity, upon which better defined and more rational principles of a more successful treatment of the disease will be based."

Recent English writers upon this subject have taken a middle ground between certain German authors, who believe in a disorder of the mental entity itself, and that much larger class who have vainly expected to connect special forms of mental aberration with pathognomonic changes of cerebral structure, and tell us that " microscopical appearances ought to be regarded more as the *effect* than the *source* of the malady" (Hitchman); that "insanity is a disease of *nervous* origin" (Munro); and that it is " a *neuralgia* of the sensory fibres of the brain" (Dewey).

"And I venture to predict," says Dr. Nichols, "that we are on the eve of the *demonstrable* discovery, that all insanity, whether of physical or moral semeiology, is proximate-

---

* Mental Maladies, p. 433.

ly owing to a derangement of the functional activity of the cerebral organ as a generator of what we are accustomed to call nerve power, nervous fluid, &c.

"That function may be exalted or depressed, through the whole or a part of the brain, as we have general mental excitement or general depression, or one or more of the infinite variety of intervening shades and forms of aberration. This purely functional derangement may, and probably not unfrequently does, run into inflammation, but they have no necessary connection, and the more furious mania may, in my opinion, exist without any more inflammatory origin or organic change than obtains in a fit of jumping' toothache, which occurs in a moment and goes in the next, without leaving any trace of its existence." *

We are thus compelled, at times, to seek the ultimate causation of insanity outside the brain.

"The special student of insanity," says Bucknill, "will do well to study the causes of delirious thought and perverted feeling, in all classes of bodily disorder where they are observable. If he studies insanity alone, he will be apt to fall into the common error of attributing its causation to some single pathological state, and his views will be as wrong as they are narrow. But, if he studies perverted feeling as occasioned by gouty or hepatic disease or loss of intellectual power, and fatal coma occasioned by suppression of the urine, and the delirium of fevers, he will be led to appreciate the full extent of blood-change in the production of purely mental affections. In the delirium of cerebritis, he will see a form of insanity undoubtedly produced by inflammation; and in delirium tremens, he will see another form of insanity, as undoubtedly produced by nervous exhaustion. He will thus be enabled to reject exclusive theories of insanity, and be prepared to admit the [truth] of the broad principle, that insanity may be occasioned by any and every pathological state which is capable of taking

* Amer. Journ. of Insanity, xi. 52.

place within the substance of the brain, however ultimately occasioned."*

The various evidences that I have now adduced should tend to convince that, as I have nowhere found expressed so clearly as by Morel, THE BRAIN IS ALWAYS THE SEAT OF INSANITY, BUT IT IS NOT ALWAYS THE SEAT OF ITS CAUSE. †

V.—Explanations of Distant Causation.

Whence else, then, can insanity arise than in the brain?

It has been supposed by some that it is generally the effect of toxæmia. This is undoubtedly at times the cause, and probably much more often than has been generally supposed. Besides the instances where its existence is self-evident, there are others. Simpson, of Edinburgh, has of late shown, with his usual masterly skill, the important relations held by that condition of the blood evinced by albuminuria, whether occasioned or not by pressure of the enlarged uterus upon the kidneys, to the existence and causation of puerperal mania.‡ Esquirol, long ago, called attention to the active effect produced by the inhalation of carbonic acid towards the induction of insanity, § and Dr Workman, in the letter from which

---

* Loc. cit., p. 349.
† Traité des Maladies Mentales, p. 69.
‡ Clinical Lectures on Diseases of Women, 1863, p. 442.
§ "We have already seen that those occupations which expose the person to

I have quoted, speaks of the tendencies towards delirium in organic pulmonary disease, and the frequency that has been observed of latent phthisis in the insane; points, both of them, that are probably to be explained by deficient elimination of carbon from the blood. It will not be strange, moreover, if it is found that in a similar manner may be interpreted much of the insanity that obtains in women, although I am not aware that this suggestion has before been made. It is well known that there is a close sympathy between the uterine and pulmonary systems, depending in part, it may be presumed, upon the varying quantities of carbon discharged by respiration and through the catamenial fluid. The evidences of this sympathy are manifold, and familiar to every gynæcologist; they are furnished alike in health and disease, explaining many types of the latter that were otherwise inexplicable, and accounting, as, for the first time, I have endeavored to show, for the fact that even were we to allow chloroform to be dangerous or deadly for the purposes of general surgery, it becomes as safe as ether, to which it is for this purpose so superior, in childbed, being here perfectly innocuous, if properly given.*

The so frequent uterine asthma, coincident or con-

---

the fumes of charcoal, predispose to insanity. We ought to add, that asphyxia by carbon, is very liable to cause dementia, and that too in its incurable form." — *Mental Maladies*, p. 54.

* Eutokia ; the employment of Anæsthetics in Childbirth, 1863, p. 20.

nected with the catamenial period, is an instance not irrelevant. I have long believed and taught, that in women the access or progress of pulmonary phthisis is frequently dependent upon and to be controlled by the menstrual condition, and I find that Dr. Workman has announced that more insane women than men die of pulmonary disease,* which is so far conclusive evidence.

"It has been noticed," I now quote from Robinson, the physician to the Bensham Asylum at Gateshead, but every one is familiar with the fact, "that among the insane generally, the circulation of the blood is feebly performed, and in melancholia more particularly, the extremities are, from this cause, cold and benumbed, while the surface of the head is often unnaturally heated. Again, in acute mania notably, and also in other recent forms of mental disorder, the quality of the blood is evidently much impaired. Our means of chemical analysis are too crude to enable us to express in scientific formulæ the precise additions and subtractions which constitute this particular cachexia. Suffice it to state that the peculiar odor and the unequivocal symptoms of disordered digestion, secretion, and excretion present in these cases, clearly show that the blood cannot be properly formed and purified, and that its condition and quality

* American Journal of Insanity, July, 1862.

must therefore be faulty. In some forms of insanity there also exists an unnatural sensibility, or irritability of the mind and nervous system, and, in a certain proportion of cases, violent mental impressions have originally induced the disease.

" Moreover, we occasionally observe in every form of mental disturbance a serious impairment of the innate vitality of the bodily tissues generally, so that a slight bruise or a degree of pressure, which, under ordinary circumstances, would produce no morbid effect whatever, will, in the insane, be followed by mortification of the parts and ultimate death." * This condition, however, is more apt to be the effect of the insanity than its cause.

On the other hand, " it should also be remembered that in many of the insane, in whom there is indisputable lesion of the understanding, the most careful scrutiny will fail to discover any disorder of the circulation, as indicated by the pulse and respiration, or of the functions of secretion and excretion, as indicated by the tongue, alvine evacuations, or the renal secretion. And, with the exception of the class of cases to be referred to, it may be safely affirmed, that among those patients whose moral nature appears to be specially invaded by disease, derangement of the physical health is almost as frequent as among those whose

---

* Prevention and Treatment of Mental Disorders, p, 152.

intellect is manifestly disordered. And the termination of cases of moral insanity in some unmistakable physical disease, as general paralysis, will not unfrequently solve any doubt which may have been felt previously, in regard to the disease of one or more of the bodily organs.

" The exceptional class we have spoken of, includes those cases of perverted moral feeling whose history extends back to their earliest infancy, and probably to congenital malformation of the brain,"* which, if not of a fœtal character, may be owing to the pressure exerted upon that organ during the latter stage of a difficult labor, or by the application of instruments during delivery.

We are not then to find in diseases of the blood, or derangement of its circulation, a causation sufficient to account for all cases of insanity which are ultimately of extra-cerebral origin. We must seek for other methods of explanation, one of which is undoubtedly the hereditary tendency so often recognized, and which may exist under very different circumstances than those ordinarily noticed. Thus, for instance, the mental disturbance may depend not merely, as I have said, upon the pressure to which the child's head has been subjected during childbirth, a pressure sufficient, in many cases, to effect its death, and in others to produce convulsions or paralysis, either

---

* Tuke, loc. cit., p. 189.

during infancy, or, perhaps, at some long subsequent period; but it may be owing to an effect produced in utero, either by some mental affection, however temporary, of the mother, just as we know such to act, during lactation, upon the nursing infant, or by some functional or organic affection of the placental or uterine system. Upon this point I could say much, but shall content myself by again presenting evidence from Dr. Tuke.

"Should it be said that disease involves a changed condition or proportion of function or structure in one or more parts of the body, it is to be observed that this change may have taken place at a period when it would escape notice, or even during fœtal life. During the latter period, diminished nutrition of the body, or diminished nutrition of one part and increased nutrition of another, may have occurred, and thus resulted in the production of an undue proportion or predominance of a function. Hypertrophy of some textures has been observed, frequently coexisting with atrophy of others, perverted nutrition being often combined with excessive or defective, and several of these different changes often occurring in succession, in consequence of the operation of the same causes. There is, indeed, during fœtal life — and we may practically widen this period, and say during that which elapses before the character is or can be observed — abundant opportunity for the influence of perverted nutrition; whether it be in the formation of cell-germs, their passage into cells, or the subsequent processes connected with the growth and organization of the tissues; or, again, whether the elements of the circulating blood be in an abnormal proportion; or, lastly, whether it be the mysterious but well-recognized principle, in virtue of which there is an hereditary predisposition to disease, which rules over and perverts the nutritive processes. Thus, in a case of what would probably be regarded as congenital moral imbecility, the mother of the patient was the subject of malignant disease of the uterus during gestation. Now it is possible that this condition of the mother interfered with the proper nutrition of the cerebral tissue of the fœtus, and was one, among other causes, which contributed to the final result. Persons born with talipes, or strabismus, owe their defect to some defect of embryo life. In like manner, during the same period of existence, the brain may undergo pathological changes which induce defective mental or moral power."*

" The emotional theory, which Bucknill believes to be the true explanation of the metaphysical nature of insanity, goes to prove only this — that emotional disturbance is the frequent source and the constant accompaniment of mental disease. It is so far practical as opposed to the theory upon which the dogmas of courts of law have been founded, that insanity is a perversion solely of the thinking faculties, but it is quite consistent with, and indeed subservient to, the opinion that the proximate cause of all mental disease is to be referred solely to the abnormal state of the brain," † the ultimate cause in many instances having to be sought also in bodily and structural change, but in parts far distant from that organ.

In justice to an earlier author, Pinel, it should be remarked that, however mistaken his views upon the pathology of insanity may have been, they had at least the merit of referring a bodily disease to a bodily origin. In the preface to the second edition of his

* Tuke, loc. cit., p. 186. † Ibid., p. 447.

work, he thus wisely expresses an emphatic condemnation of metaphysical theories on this point: —

"The most difficult part of natural history is, without doubt, the art of well observing internal diseases, and of distinguishing them by their proper characters. But mental alienation presents new and diverse difficulties and obstacles to surmount, either in the unusual gestures and tumultuous agitations which it occasions, or in a kind of disordered and incoherent chatter, or in a repulsive or savage exterior. If one desires to account for the phenomena observed, one has to fear another rock — that of intermingling metaphysical discussions and divagations of ideology with a science of facts."*

He goes still further, and with an acumen remarkable in view of the limited method of diagnosis then known, he foreshadows the great theory of a frequent pelvic origin, for he refers the primitive seat of mania "to the region of the stomach and intestines, from whence, as from a centre, the disorder of the understanding is propagated by a species of irradiation. A feeling of constriction, &c., manifests itself in these parts, soon followed by a disorder and trouble of ideas."† In that day, it will be remembered, the methods, by which at the present time the differential diagnosis of most of the diseases of the abdomen is so clearly and so easily established, were in practice almost wholly unknown.

We have thus been brought to the doctrine that mental disturbance may be occasioned secondarily

---

* Tuke, p. 394.   † Ibid., p. 393.

and reflexly, by sympathy with disturbances of other organs than the brain. Let us listen upon the general subject, to Dr. Bucknill.

"That the organ of the mind is thrown into diseased action by sympathy with, that is, by suffering with, other diseased or injured parts, is scarcely less certain than that the stomach, the heart, or the spinal marrow are so affected. The modus operandi of this cause of disease is by no means clearly intelligible, either in relation to the brain or to other organs; the explanations usually offered being little more than diversified verbal formularies of the fact. Thus, when we say that the irritation of the cervix uteri is reflected upon the stomach, occasioning vomiting and distress in that organ, we come no nearer to an explanation of the mode of action than when we say that the stomach sympathizes with, or suffers in conjunction with, or in consequence of, irritation of the organ first affected. And, in like manner, when we say that the brain suffers sympathetically with the uterus or stomach, we use a mere verbal formula for the colligation of two facts, with the intimate nature of whose connection we are wholly unacquainted. The knowledge which we actually possess on this subject may, in general terms, be thus stated: the most important organs of the body are liable to be thrown into states of functional disturbance by irritation or injury of other, and frequently of distant parts. The liability to this disturbance depends, in the first place, upon what is called constitutional irritability, or a state of the system in which slight causes of nervous action produce great effects; and, in the second place, upon the intimate connection of the organ secondarily affected, with the nervous system, and its liability to be thrown into disorder by any alteration or disturbance in the state of that system. Any premature attempts to explain this important pathological fact by hypothesis, respecting nervous currents, or the exhaustion of nervous power, seem at present rather likely to obscure than elucidate the matter. We may, however, come one step nearer to the view of the fact, by considering all sympathetic disturbance as taking place in the nervous system itself; and in viewing the functional disturbance of secreting and other organs, as merely the expression of abnormal states of the nerves in those organs. Strictly speaking, therefore, sympathetic vomiting or palpitation is as purely a nervous phenomenon as loss of consciousness or convulsions; and the latter, as mental excitement or delusion.

"In early life, the cerebro-mental functions are more intimately connected with those of the spinal system than at subsequent periods, and distant irritations are more frequent and efficient causes of mental disturbance in the infant than in the adult. Delirium and coma are, in children, frequently produced by intestinal irritation. In the adult, in comparison with convulsions, delirium is so rarely a consequence of simple irritation, that it furnishes one strong proof that the brain proper exercises its functions with great independence of the excito-motory or spinal system. The most frequent and unquestionable instances of cerebral disturbance from distant irritation or sympathy, are afforded in epilepsy and hysteria. In both of these diseases the paroxysm is compounded of disturbance both of the cerebral and spinal functions; but during the interval, cerebral disturbance alone is frequently present, and in the paroxysm itself it is never wanting. In epilepsy, especially, is this the case; for loss of consciousness, which is the primary and leading feature of the paroxysm, is the most serious and profound indication of cerebral disturbance, no less, in fact, than the temporary abnegation of all cerebral function. In hysteria, loss of consciousness is of less certain occurrence, although sometimes it is doubtless complete. In the interval of hysteria, however, cerebral disturbance is not less marked than in epilepsy. The emotions are perverted, and even delirium is by no means uncommon. Now both of these diseases are frequently but the expression of sympathy with irritation of distant parts of the nervous system. The one is produced by irritation of the nerves of the uterus and its appendages, and the other by the irritation of almost any portion of the peripheral nerves, by worms in the intestines, renal calculus, painful injuries, and diseases of the limbs, &c. Therefore these diseases present unquestionable instances of mental disturbance, occasioned by sympathy of the brain with irritation of the distant nerves; of the central organ of the system, suffering in its noblest functions, in sympathy with some fibres of its peripheral extension.

"The most probable explanation of these sympathetic disorders is, that injury to one part of the nervous system interferes with the processes of secondary nutrition taking place in other parts. The rapidity with which they occur may. at first sight, seem adverse to this view; for instance, in the case related by Dr. Gooch, and so familiar to psychologists, where Dr. Denman passed a ligature round a polypus of the fundus of the uterus; as soon as he tightened it, he produced pain and vomiting. As soon as the ligature was slackened, the pain ceased; but whenever he attempted to tighten it, the pain and vomiting returned. The ligature was left on, but loose. The patient died about six weeks afterwards, and, on opening the body, it was found that the uterus was inverted, and that the ligature had included the inverted portion. Sympathetic disturbances of the functions of the brain are, in some instances, scarcely less rapidly occasioned, or capable of receiving more immediate relief. Thus the irritation of a cutting tooth will sometimes produce in a child delirium and coma; and the removal of the irritation, by incision of the inflamed gum, will remove the symptoms almost as speedily as in the examples above quoted. But when it is considered that the processes of secondary nutrition are those upon which the functions of all organs immediately depend, and that any interference with these processes must necessarily and immediately disturb the normal course of the functions, the short interval which is frequently observed to exist between the production of irritation and its sympathetic consequences will present no difficulty to the theory which explains the latter in the manner here suggested. In our present state of ignorance of the manner in which influences are communicated from one part of the nervous system to other parts, it is impossible to explain how the processes of secondary nutrition in the nervous structure are interfered with in distant parts thereof. But this difficulty scarcely diminishes the probability that the explanation offered is the true one; and, indeed, only presents one of those imperfect links in reasoning, which the immaturity of physiological science renders of such constant occurrence in all departments of medicine. The operation of remedies is consistent with this view of sympathetic disturbance, since those narcotic substances which retard the processes of waste and repair in the nervous system afford the most efficient means of preventing the nervous function from suffering in consequence of peripheral nervous injury. Moreover, this view of pathological sympathy is consistent with the only rational view of physiological sympathy. Secretions are the result of secondary nutrition. Many secretions are normally excited by the irritation of nerves more or less distant; that of the mamma, for instance, of the testis, and, to some extent, of the gastric glands. Here, then, at least, are processes of secondary nutrition, energetically influenced by the irritation of distant nerves."[*]

Marshall Hall himself could scarcely have afforded us a juster and more thorough argument for all the effects I have claimed, of pelvic agencies as ultimately causing insanity in women, than the remarks above given.

It has been argued that those of us who see in reflex action an explanation of what would be otherwise inexplicable anomalies, must be in error on the ground that, by allowing a distant lesion ever to produce disturbance of the brain, we ought always to

[*] Loc. cit., pp. 382–385.

find an identical effect from a similar cause. The fallacy of such an expectation has been commented upon by Dr. Williams in the following language, equally applicable to congestion and other morbid conditions of the brain: —

"Congestion of the liver is sometimes accompanied by pain or tenderness; sometimes it is without either. Congestion of the stomach sometimes causes gastralgia, nausea, and vomiting, with altered appetite; but these symptoms are often absent when the amount of disease of the liver, or the heart, and the subsequent occurrence of hæmatemesis, leave no doubt that the stomach was congested. The same remark is applicable to the kidneys, the uterus, the brain, and other organs." *

On the other hand, that in cases where mental disturbance is thus induced, it should often be extreme, varying alike in its type, its symptomatic characters, and its degree of intensity, is only what should *à priori* have been expected. Dr. Bucknill has clearly recognized this fact, and admits that the analogy from an organ whose function is simple, to one whose function is so complex as that of the brain, can afford but a slight insight into the effect of similar pathological conditions in the two instances. Of the abdominal and thoracic organs, the stomach is that whose functions are the least simple. Its muscular movements are as ingeniously adapted to an end as are those of the heart; they are even more complicated and less mechanical. In addition to this, the functions

* Principles of Medicine.

of secretion and absorption, discharged by its several sets of glands, add to the complexity of its duties. Congestion, as we have seen, causes irregular excitement or depression of all its functions, nervous, muscular, and secretive; yet, compared with the brain, how few and simple are its duties. The functions of the organ of the mind are more numerous than those of all other parts of the body put together; nor less distinct in themselves and inter-distinct in their action. Consequently, any pathological state which destroys their equilibrium, producing irregular depression of some functions, with irregular excitement of others, must cause a wider and more intricate range of anomalies than is observable in a similar state of the more simple organs.*

It is necessary to distinguish the distant affections which cause insanity from those that merely accompany or result from mental disturbance. I have already referred to Dr. Workman's estimate of the frequency and importance in the insane, of pulmonary phthisis, here so often latent or unnoticed, even to its extreme stages. The physician of the Devon Asylum would explain this and similar affections in the insane as follows:—

"Diseases of the lungs occur in the insane in all their varieties. They are frequently latent from the absence of cough, and the patient's absorption of mind preventing com-

* Loc. cit., p. 359.

plaint. The absence of cough in serious pulmonary disease is very peculiar. In dementia, it arises partly from torpor of the excito-motory system, partly from loss of attention; from the same cause, in fact, as the frequent dirty habits of the insane. In mania, it arises from the attention being intensely pre-occupied by the vivid ideas and delusions which absorb the mind. We have seen many patients in advanced stages of phthisis, who were never heard to cough so long as they were under the influence of maniacal excitement. When this underwent a temporary diminution, they were greatly troubled with cough, which was again arrested by the recurrence of excitement. The continuance of colliquative diarrhœa and perspiration, and of emaciation, proved that there was no halt in the progress of the disease, as the absence of cough has led authors erroneously to suppose. The torpor of the nervous system in dementia leads to another peculiarity in the lung and in some other bodily diseases of the insane, namely, the absence of irritative or symptomatic fever; and hence it happens, that in a demented person whose strength is unimpaired, and whose constitution is tolerably good, diseases will obtain a high degree of development, with symptoms so few or obscure as to be incredible to the general physician. It is on this account that the numerous sloughing sores to which general paralytics are liable, produce so little suffering or constitutional irritation. We have known the stomach disorganized by cancer, without the patient complaining of any pain until a few days before death, when perforation took place. The only case of true carditis we ever saw, occurred in an insane person who complained of no pain, and in whose heart disease was only suspected twenty-four hours before death, in consequence of the failure of the pulse. This peculiarity in the intercurrent diseases of the insane should teach the physician to observe with watchful anxiety every physical indication from which he can derive knowledge of the attack of disease before it is so advanced as to be beyond control. Pulmonary gangrene is more common among the insane than the sane; but not to the same extent here as at Vienna, where it contributes largely to asylum mortality."*

To my own mind, it would be more scientific and in accordance with facts to explain the non-appreciation of pain in the insane by a true state of general or local anæsthesia, a temporary and intermittent, or confirmed and permanent, paralysis of the nerves of sensation, local and limited or general as this may be, than to attribute it merely to lack of notice of the suffering, in consequence of pre-engagement or preoccupation of the mind. That I am correct would seem to be shown, moreover, by the curious fact that there is often absent in the insane the febrile excitement and reaction, both nervous and arterial, that usually attend physical accident or disease. That intervals may occur, in which the patient becomes acutely sensible of bodily anguish, only implies that æsthesia or even hyperæsthesia may succeed to local or general anæsthesia, just as undue mental activity may at times alternate with apathy or even dementia itself.

VI.—Causation of Insanity often Pelvic in Women.

I have claimed that while there are affections of many organs in the body in both sexes, that underlie

---

* Loc. cit., p. 433.

insanity, being in reality its cause, and the foundation upon which it rests, in women there is a depth beyond — a source of excitation not existing, practically, in man; for, allowing every latitude to the influence of the sexual system in the male, it must be allowed that in him the genital apparatus is merely subsidiary, and playing but an occasional and comparatively a very insignificant part in its relations to the general economy.

In woman, the case is very different. Not only is she subject to a host of diseases peculiar to her sex, to which we find neither homologue nor analogue in man, but they are capable of so modifying herself as entirely to change her natural disposition and character. In health, we find her still obedient to a special law. The subject here also, we might even say the victim, of periodicity, her life is one perpetual change, and these changes even are still again subdivided.

The uterus and appendages that, in the female embryo, while yet unborn, were being developed *pari passu* with the other organs of the body, become at birth arrested in their growth; without other change than a slight and disproportionate enlargement in size, they remain in their fœtal condition until puberty occurs. The child has now become a maiden. Immediately the emotions, desires, and passions that, though latent, have been gradually foreshadowing themselves, are now established, unrecognized though they may be by the girl herself; yet, like the smouldering fires of a volcano, ready to burst forth at any exciting moment. The short space of a lunar month is henceforward the field, for many years, of a triple change — preparation for ovulation, the discharge of a germ fit for impregnation, rest and recuperation. The instinctive yearning for the other sex, and its gratification in the excitement of coitus, the culmination of sexual congress in effectual impregnation, are surely of no little import; as they are affairs of constantly recurring occurrence, both in the married and in many of the unmarried, unless, as is too often the case, they are interfered with by preventive or subversive measures, which may but increase their effects upon the woman's system by making them prejudicial rather than, as otherwise, of benefit. Pregnancy with its varying fortunes, childbed and lactation, and, finally, the grand climacteric, supervene, and a return to the second sexual childhood, which, though barren of further fruit to the womb, is yet by no means past desire and attempts at its gratification, or past uterine disease and its many dangers: with this the scene is closed.

To man, these changes, these excitements, this special work, these diseases, these dangers, are all unknown. Why, then, is it called preposterous to seek in her sex the abstract fundamental influence impressed upon every woman, even while an infant in her mother's womb, the solution of much to which otherwise we have no key? Van Helmont was not far wrong when he contended that woman was what she is, in health, in character, in her charms, alike of body, mind, and soul, because of her womb alone.

Nor am I so far wrong, I candidly believe, in attributing the major part, not all, of her characteristics in disease, mental as well as bodily, also to this self-same womb. Just as we have special diseases of the pelvic organs in the female, so we may have functional diseases of the brain, of many and deceptive types, excited in her thereby; and just as we may have other disease in woman, whether general in its character or of other than uterine localization, pulmonary, cardiac, renal, or hepatic, as the case may be, idiopathic in its inception, yet materially modified by the influence of the sexual system, even so there may exist states of mental disturbance in which we may recognize an originality of causation in the brain itself, but yet such an effect from a special physiological or pathological condition of the uterus or ovaries that may be present, as to require special examination, special consideration, and special treatment. To the gynæcological expert, these facts will be self-evident. I have found that to some psychological experts they have not been so. As my object is merely to change to a more rational system the present private and public treatment of so many of the most interesting of patients, now practically untreated at all, I shall again present the testimony of psychologists rather than my own. In my previous writings I have contended that the principles to which I had called attention have long been known, though in practice constantly unappreciated or forgotten. I shall now go farther, and by the testimony presented, which is but a little fraction of that I now have at hand, show, as I think, conclusively, that in longer refusing for the female insane that study, special examination, and treatment, without which, in all other forms of disease, women cannot be properly cared for, any person laying claim to the honorable office of physician must be deemed guilty of gross neglect, blindness from too great conservatism, or inhumanity. This is strong language: it is not intended as personal, however. I am but working for a general principle in one of the many fields of its application, and in behalf of the sex, to the alleviation of whose sufferings some of us are devoting our lives. Should controversies be attempted to be forced upon me, as has already been the case in the discussion of this question, it is to the good sense and wisdom of the profession that I shall again appeal.

I cannot do better, at this point of our inquiry, than introduce the testimony of a gentleman at present, or very lately, connected with the Utica Asylum.

"When we contemplate the reproductive system, whether

in health or disease," says Dr. Kellogg, "in its relations to the cerebral system and to psychology, we are forcibly struck with the paucity and imperfection of our knowledge. The recorded facts which bear upon the reciprocal influence of these systems are widely scattered, and the attempt to collect, digest, and systematize them, and make the necessary scientific deductions, would be a work of some importance.*

"The influence of excessive and unnatural excitement of the sexual organs upon the mental faculties," he continues, "has long been recognized. In tables setting forth the supposed causes of insanity, this has long occupied a prominent place; and though its influence as a cause of insanity has no doubt been overrated (or misinterpreted, in the absence of physical examinations in women, — H. R. S.), still it is undoubtedly great.† Of the probable causes of derangement in three hundred and sixty-six cases of insanity, occurring in both sexes, — as recorded in the report of the superintendent of the New York State Lunatic Asylum, for the year 1852, — eighty-seven, or nearly one fourth of the whole number of cases, are reported to have arisen from causes directly connected with the reproductive system. In the report of the superintendent of the same institution for the year 1853, of the supposed causes of insanity in four hundred and twenty-four cases, one hundred and seventeen, or more than one fourth, appear to have had direct connection with some disturbance of the sexual organs. In the able and interesting report of Dr. Gray to the managers of this institution, for 1853, of three hundred and ninety cases, seventy-two are supposed to have had some direct connection with derangement of these organs. From the above, it would appear that in nearly one fourth of all the cases of insanity, occurring in both sexes, the disturbance of the generative organs was so marked as to be regarded as a primary cause of the mental derangement.

---

* Considerations on the Reciprocal Influence of the Physical Organization and Mental Manifestations. — Amer. Journal of Insanity, April, 1856, p. 305

† See the testimony of the late Dr. Brigham, in the Philips' Will case. — Amer. Journal of Insanity, vol. vi. p. 182.

"Whether the primary cause in these cases had its seat in the cerebral or the generative system, is a question no less interesting than difficult of solution, and one which could only be determined by an attentive consideration of the history of the cases reported, and a close observance of the true sequence of the symptoms in each, and, whether the primary link in the chain of morbid sympathies had its seat in the one system or the other, it is none the less important in relation to the reciprocal influence of the two.

"As the functions of the reproductive system are far more important and intricate in the female than in the male economy, and as the pathological disturbances are, as a natural consequence of this, more frequent and interesting, we are, as a matter of course, to look to the female generative system for the most important illustrations of the sympathetic disturbances and reciprocal influences dependent upon these pathological lesions. Hence, all the diseases which affect the female generative system have, at one time or another, been brought forward as causes of insanity. Even its most natural function, that of gestation, does, in some cases, by the peculiar change wrought in the female economy, and the train of inexplicable symptoms which result, give rise to insanity; and there are cases on record, of females who have been positively insane during the whole of each period of utero-gestation, but who recovered their mental health and strength soon after delivery. The cases in which some slight mental or moral disturbance during gestation has been observed are numerous; there are many on record, and every experienced practitioner is able, no doubt, to recall to mind such slight disturbances.

"The influence which the menstrual function, even when performed apparently in a healthy manner, exercises upon the mental faculties and moral feelings of some females is exceedingly interesting to the intelligent and philosophical observer. In certain abnormal states of this function the influence is still more apparent. I have been told by intelligent females, accustomed to analyze their own feelings, that they felt far less mental energy during this state than in the intervals, and that they possessed far less control over the moral feelings than at other times, were more easily excited, and that the most trifling circumstances, which at other times would pass unheeded, have, in spite of every effort, greatly disturbed their equanimity. In some whom I have known, of a nervous, excitable temperament, their whole character appeared changed during the menstrual period, and from being cheerful, kind, firm, patient, and decided, they became morose, taciturn, wayward, fidgety, and impatient, frequently manifesting a certain nervous irritability bordering on hysteria, and were sometimes overcome by paroxysms of that interesting affection.

"The changes which take place in the mental and moral faculties about the time of puberty, are in both sexes very interesting, particularly so with the female. These have been frequently alluded to by medical writers, as attendant upon a fuller development and higher manifestations of vitality in the sexual organs. During these changes the nervous system exhibits increased susceptibility and sensibility; and not only the whole frame, but also the mental manifestations, present greater activity of development." "The mind," says Dr. Copland, "acquires extended powers of emotion and passion, and the imagination becomes more lively. If, on the other hand, the uterine organs continue undeveloped, and the menstrual discharge does not appear, the mind is dull, weak, or depressed, and the emotions and passions are imperfect or altogether absent." *

"The young female," resumes Dr. Kellogg, "who, up to the time of these changes, has appeared, comparatively speaking, a non-sexual being in her intercourse with her companions, playing in childlike innocence and unrestrained freedom with the opposite sex as with her own, — ignorant and unconscious of the powers within her, which are soon to be awakened from their slumbers, — begins, as she now approaches the verge of womanhood, to be animated with feelings and desires to which she was before a complete stranger, and which she regards with a deep interest as the

* Dictionary of Medicine, art. Menstruation, vol. ii. p. 959.

forerunners of something, she scarcely knows what, which she feels inclined to cherish, yet shrinks from, as though she knew not whether they were of good or evil omen.

"In her intercourse with her former playmates of the opposite sex, there appears gradually to have dawned upon her an interesting shyness and maidenly reserve. Expressions which before conveyed no meaning to her pure mind, and which even now are but partially understood, are yet sufficiently so to tinge her cheek, and cause her to shrink back instinctively, as from some foul and pestilential presence. Her likes and dislikes are stronger, and rendered more apparent to those around her. In short, the physical changes brought about in a limited period of time in the sexual system have wrought a complete change in the mental and moral character of the young girl, and this period of transition terminates in that of complete womanhood, with all its desires and its aspirations, its hopes and its fears, its joys and its sorrows.

"But it is in connection with the various diseases incident to the female generative system that we are to look for the more curious illustrations of this cerebral sympathy. The abnormal mental state of many patients laboring under hysteria, menorrhagia, dysmenorrhœa, amenorrhœa, and the affections intimately associated with uterine derangement, has long been observed by medical men." "In at least three cases out of four," says Dr. Francis, "I have found hysteria associated with uterine derangement, and the restoration of the menstrual function to its healthy state has proved the precursor of the removal of the hysterical annoyance." Hysteria, again, may manifest itself chiefly by disorder of the mental faculties, and the moral feelings and emotions. "The mental affections," observes Dr. Copland, "connected with hysteria may be referred, 1. to certain states of monomania, among which excited desire, amounting in some cases to nymphomania, may be enumerated; 2. to ecstasies and mental excitement, in some cases of a religious nature, in others of different descriptions; 3. to a state of somnambulism; 4. to a form of delirium, generally of a lively character, with which various hysterical symptoms are often conjoined; 5. to various delusions, generally of a hypochondriacal kind, to which the patient may become subject or even the victim, owing to the indulgence she may meet with from imprudently kind relatives; and, 6. to a desire to feign various diseases, sometimes of an anomalous or singular form."*

The subjoined remarks of this same acute and philosophical physician are so apposite that we cannot resist the temptation to transcribe them in this connection.

"Hysterical females," says he, "are not merely capricious or whimsical, but they often become enthusiastic for a time in the pursuit of an object, or in cherishing an emotion by which they have been excited. In many such cases the nervous excitement and vascular turgescence of the uterine organs determine the character of the mental disorder, elevating certain of the moral sentiments, or of the intellectual manifestations, to a state of extravagance, passing in some instances into delusion or monomania. Many cases of puerperal mania are merely extremes of the hysterical disorder of the moral and intellectual powers or states of the mind. All these more extreme forms of mental affection are observed only where, in connection with much local or uterine irritation, there is great deficiency of nervous energy generally, and of mental power in particular; or where, with such deficiency, there has been much injudicious culture or perversion, or improper excitement of the imagination. Females sometimes become passionately attached to an object, and this passion may advance even to nymphomania or monomania.

"The hypochondriacal feelings, the desire to deceive, or to simulate various diseases, or the delusions which sometimes possess the minds of hysterical females, may be classed with the foregoing, as requiring a similar plan of treatment. In

* Loc. citat., vol. ii. p. 321.

all of them the intentions of cure are to remove irritation or vascular turgescence of the uterine organs; to improve the general health; to strengthen the nervous system; to calm the imagination; and to guide the moral impulses of the patient. The most efficient, however, of these means are not likely to be adopted by the patient. Few will resort daily to the shower-bath, or even occasionally to terebinthinate enemata, or submit to a course of tonics, or to a suitable regimen, &c., while they believe their health but little affected. Even when the hysterical disorder is of a very painful kind, the variability or capricious state of the patient's mind leads her to run from one physician to another, before opportunity of administering aid is afforded to any. At last, the most notorious charlatans, particularly those who excite the body through the mind or the mind through the body, the animal magnetizers, the homœopathists, the St. John Longs of rubbing celebrity, and the Campbells of celestial-bed notoriety, fix her attention. At such medical bagnios there is something promising gratification as well as excitement, and at such places hysterical as well as hypochondriacal patients 'most do congregate.' *

"When we pass from the consideration of the influence of the reproductive system upon the cerebral, to take a view of the influence of the latter upon the former, we enter upon an inquiry possessing as profound an interest as any in the whole domain of science; and here, again, as before, we have to look to the female economy for the most interesting facts and phenomena illustrative of this mysterious and inexplicable sympathy. The results of this influence, if we allow ourselves to believe the statements and receive as evidence what is brought forward as fact in illustration of it, are, indeed, sometimes most extraordinary; and the unmistakable evidence of this, which is from time to time presented to the medical observer, is sometimes so curious as to make him pause before rejecting, as the workings of a morbid imagination, the statements which are sometimes made by intelligent females, whose veracity we cannot doubt,

* Copland, loc. citat., vol. ii. p. 337.

and whose motives for deceiving us we are unable to discover.

"There are few physicians of experience who will not be able to call to mind some extraordinary statements made to them by females in reference to this sympathy, which at the time, no doubt, merely called forth a smile of incredulity or surprise at what was then regarded as the result of superstition, or of a morbid imagination, but which, in after hours, has been seized upon as food for reflection." *

To these remarks of Dr. Kellogg, there would be little need of adding, had they but been practically accepted and acted upon. Such, however, has not been the case. Nearly ten years have elapsed since their publication, and, as yet, in the reports of no asylum do we find a change, either in the method of tabulating cases, of specifying causes, or of treatment. The organ of psychologists in this country, the American Journal of Insanity, generally so ably conducted, in which Dr. Kellogg's paper appeared, and which emanates from the asylum with which he is connected, still ignores the conclusions he had advanced, as shown alike in its editorial papers and in its comments, or absence of comments, upon those by others, admitted to its pages. I need adduce but a single instance. Sir William Hamilton, in his celebrated work upon metaphysics, makes use of the following language: "A fact striking in itself," he says, "and not without significance in relation to the present inquiry, is this, that these intruders" (parasitic animals

---

* American Journal of Insanity, April, 1856, pp. 306-10.

of various kinds, worms in every loathsome diversity, reptiles armed with fangs, crawlers of a hundred feet, &c., &c.), "infest the (frontal) sinuses of women." This statement, so strange and astonishing as regards its application to most women, sane or insane, was reproduced in the Journal referred to, by a reviewer of Hamilton, but ten years ago, without a word of contradiction.*

While a single fact like the above can take place, a single assertion of that character pass unchallenged alike by the Journal and the profession at large, it cannot be argued either that the conclusions presented in this report are generally known and acted upon, or that the investigation is one without a very plain and practical end.

The notion that her sex plays an important part in the causation of insanity in women, is by no means a modern one. Like many of the most valuable theories of medicine, it dates back to remotest antiquity.

Aretæus, of Cappadocia, held that a frequent cause of mania was to be found in suppression of the menses, or difficulty in their establishment in young women, who needed only this condition of marriage.*

Soranus enumerates, among other causes, the long continued use of medicines that excite the genital organs in women, and the suppression of their periodical

---

* American Journal of Insanity, June, 1860, p. 255.
† Trélat: Récherches Historiques sur la Folie, 1839, p. 12.

discharge.* Before the expedition of the Argonauts, and before Hippocrates, it is said that the daughters of King Prœtus, whose savage lowings† remind one of certain historical and modern epidemics of insanity complicated with hysteria, were cured by means of hellebore, which was then supposed to exercise a peculiar influence upon the uterus.‡ The theory of pelvic causation, like all others, however good, did not even at that early period escape criticism. Cœlius Aurelianus, for instance, affirmed that women were less subject to insanity than men; but his reviewers and admirers of more modern times, and at the present day, however they undertake to explain the fact, yet think that he was mistaken. This statement is true of Esquirol, Copland, Brown, and many others, some of whom I shall hereafter quote. Thus, Dr. Haslam has averred, speaking of England, that " in our own climate, women are more frequently afflicted with insanity than men."

On the other hand, to bring this disputed question down to the present moment, Dr. Thurnam, in his paper upon the relative liability of the two sexes to insanity, expresses himself as follows: —

"Having thus shown that in the principal hospitals for the insane in these kingdoms, the proportion of men admitted is nearly always higher, and, in many instances, much

---

* Morel: Traité des Maladies Mentales, p. 4.
† " Prœtides implerunt falsis mugitibus agros." Ibid., p. 19.
‡ Griffith: Medical Botany, p. 86.

higher than that of women, and as we know that the proportion of men in the general population, particularly at those ages when insanity most usually occurs, is decidedly less than that of women, we can have no ground for doubting that men are actually more liable to disorders of the mind than women." *

Dr. Bucknill, also, is of opinion that it is clearly proved that, in general, fewer women become insane than men.†

Upon this side the water, this question of the comparative liability of males and females to insanity, has been carefully investigated by Dr. Edward Jarvis, of Dorchester, in a paper published in the Journal of Insanity several years since. He also has arrived at the conclusion that males are somewhat more liable to insanity than females.

There are, it will be perceived, several very different questions here involved, as the following: —

1. Do more women, abstractly, than men, become insane?

2. Do more women become insane, in proportion to the number of each sex existing in a given hospital, city, state, or country?

3. Do more women than men become insane from sexual causes?

The latter question, it will be perceived, is the only one that concerns us in the present inquiry. It is to the two former, however, that attention has gen-

* Quarterly Journal of the Statistical Society of London, December, 1844.
† Loc. cit., p. 245.

erally been given. As the attempt at their solution, though this must evidently be almost impossible, has been made, I will give it a moment's notice. Dr. Bucknill has admitted that there are many points that observers have practically lost sight of.

"Sufficient care," he says, "does not appear to have been taken to ascertain the relative number of males and females in the general population, a point obviously necessary to determine, before any just conclusion can be drawn as to the relative liability of the sexes to insanity. Writers upon the subject have found the existing number of female lunatics greater than that of the males, and hence, have arrived at the conclusion that the female sex is more subject to insanity than the male. Dr. Thurnam, however, has pointed out this source of fallacy, as well as that which arises from the fact that the mortality of insane men exceeds that of insane women by fifty per cent. Hence it is obvious that Esquirol erred, in comparing the existing instead of the occurring cases of insanity in the male and female sexes. If, in our asylums, women live longer than men, they will of course proportionately accumulate."

"In order that the comparison of the occurring cases be a strictly accurate one," observes Thurnam, "the proportions of the two sexes at the several ages, attacked with insanity for the first time, should be compared with the proportions in which the two sexes at the same ages exist in the community in which such cases occur. The nearest approximation to this method which we have the means of employing is, by assuming that the proportions of men and women admitted into public institutions during extensive periods represent — as, on the whole, they probably do represent — the cases which occur for the first time."

"From an examination of a table prepared by this writer, it was ascertained that, in twenty-four of the thirty-two asylums, which it comprises, there had been a decided excess of men in the numbers admitted. In many British asylums, the excess amounts to twenty-five, thirty, and even forty per cent., and, in the whole number of thirty-two asylums, there is an average excess on the side of the male sex of thirteen and seven one hundredths per cent. In the nine English county asylums contained in the table, the excess amounts to twelve per cent.

"From the same tables, it appears that, in the asylums of the metropolis, the proportion of females admitted is much greater than in the provinces. This appears to be in part accounted for by there being a considerable excess per cent. (thirteen per cent. at all ages, and nineteen per cent. at all ages above twenty) of women over men in the metropolis.* Hence, the experience of Bethlem and St. Luke's led Dr. Webster to the conclusion, that no doubt can exist regarding the greater frequency of mental alienation among females than males. Dr. Thurnam appears to regard it as probable, that the statistics of insanity in France resemble in this particular those of London, although, as has been pointed out, the method of inquiry adopted by Esquirol was vicious.

"Jarvis has shown," continues Bucknill, "that the causes of insanity which act upon males are more extensive than those which act upon females, and has added that the above statement, in regard to the liability of the sexes, must vary with different nations, different periods of the world, and different habits of the people.

"It would be difficult to establish that the female sex is intrinsically less susceptible to the causes of insanity than the male, since the former is less exposed to those causes than the latter; at least, to establish the greater intrinsic liability of females, it must be shown that they are exposed to the predisposing and exciting causes of insanity to as great an extent as males." †

* On the other hand, in some parts of this country, in Massachusetts for instance, the excess of women is much greater than in London, being estimated of late at fifty per cent., or even higher; and yet there seems to be no proportionate excess of female admissions at asylums.

† Loc. cit.; p. 245. This last sentence is expressive only of Bucknill's opinion; I think it will appear that women are exposed constantly to the action of these causes to a greater extent than are men.

In this connection, as in many others, it must not be forgotten that the statistics of the insane, whether derived from hospitals or from the general population, are very liable to be faulty or to give rise to erroneous conclusions. I shall subsequently give evidence to this effect, and the opinions of Luther V. Bell and others; here merely asking, —

"What can be the value of medical statistics in any disease, under which sixty per cent. of the entire cases must be left unaccounted for? Probably too, not five out of twenty of the assigned causes are justly chargeable with the mental disease ascribed to them." *

In the present instance, writers seem to have lost sight of the facts that in almost all countries more males than females are born; that this percentage of excess, which would be very much greater were all the males that are conceived born living, is to a certain extent kept down by the number of boys who die in infancy and during childhood in consequence of various affections to which the comparatively larger size of the head in the male fœtus has given rise, from the greater pressure to which it was necessarily subjected during parturition; † and that in this

---

* Workman: Report of the Provincial Lunatic Asylum at Toronto, 1863, p. 5.

† Dr. Simpson, in his memoirs upon the sex of the child as a cause of difficulty and danger in human parturition, has shown conclusively, that —

1. Of the mothers that die under parturition and its immediate consequences, a much greater portion have given birth to male than female children.

2. Among labors presenting morbid complications and difficulties, the child is much oftener male than female.

3. Among the children of the mothers that die from labor or its consequences,

same excess of cerebral compression, is undoubtedly to be found an efficient cause of insanity in man in after life. This point does not appear to have been before observed. It has also been forgotten that males everywhere, save perhaps in the most crowded cities, are much more likely than women to be carried from home and the care of relatives to the seclusion of an asylum; that in women, the attacks are more seldom persistent, more frequently intermittent, paroxysmal, periodical, and therefore more likely to be endured by friends, and to be more constantly looked upon as merely hysterical, nervous or feigned, while no one at all familiar with the subject would undertake to prove, as Bucknill has supposed

---

a larger proportion of those that are still-born are male than female; and, on the contrary, of those that are born alive a larger proportion are female than male.

4. Of still-born children, a larger proportion are male than female.

5. Of the children that die during the actual progress of parturition, the number of males is much greater than the number of females.

6. Of the children born alive, more males than females are seen to suffer from the morbid states and injuries resulting from parturition.

7. More male than female children die in the earliest period of infancy, and the disproportion between the mortality of the two sexes gradually diminishes from birth onwards, until some time subsequently.

8. Of the children that die in utero and before the commencement of labor, as large a proportion are females as males.

9. In laborious labor with the head presenting, in proportion as the order of labor rises in difficulty, the amount of male births rises in number.

10. Of the morbid accidents that are liable to happen in connection with the third stage of labor, after the head has passed the brim of the pelvis, as many take place with female as with male births.

11. More dangers and deaths occur both to mothers and children in first than in subsequent labors.

12. The average duration of labor is longer with male than with female children. — *Obstetric Works.* Edited by Drs. Priestley and H. R. Storer. Edinburgh edition, i. p. 394.

possible, that women are intrinsically *less* susceptible to the same causes of insanity that affect men. On the contrary, we would claim that these very productive and efficient causes do act, so far as women are exposed to them, and a thousand-fold more besides.

It has been supposed that moral influences, and those purely mental in their character, have exercised an important part in the causation of insanity. In the case of women, in the absence of a predisposition to insanity by inheritance, I believe that these moral causes seldom efficiently act unless in the presence of physical disturbance.

Be this as it may, much attention has been paid by psychologists to the classification of these alleged moral excitations. Thus Tuke, from an analysis of some thirty thousand cases, admitted into a large number of asylums in England, France, and America, found that among them domestic troubles or grief stand first in the list in every instance; next in order, religious anxiety or excitement; then disappointed affections, political and other excitements, fear and fright; and lastly, excessive study and wounded feelings, as impaired self-love, etc.* There is, of course, no doubt that men are more exposed than women to political excitement and the harassing anxieties of business; but these we find Esquirol considering as more than counterbalanced by the

* Manual, p. 258.

vices of female education; the preference given to acquirements purely ornamental; the reading of romances, from which arises a precocious activity of the intellect and premature desires, together with ideas of an imaginary excellence that can never be realized; the frequenting of plays and society; the abuse of music and the want of occupation—these, he thinks, are causes sufficient to make insanity most frequent among women.*

Dr. Conolly, of the Hanwell Asylum, but reiterates this opinion when he says that—

"All who have peculiar opportunities of ascertaining the mental habits of insane persons of the educated classes well know that, with some exceptions, their previous studies and pursuits appear to have been superficial and desultory, and often frivolous; the condition of the female mind, especially of the minds of those who are to be the mothers of another generation, is, even in the highest classes, too often more deplorable still. Not only is it most rare to find them familiar with the best authors of their own country, but most common to find that they have never read a really good author, either in their own or in any other language; and that the few accomplishments possessed by them have been taught for display in society, and not for solace in quieter hours. All this has been said before, and often, and in vain. But there is a frequent perversion of intellectual exercise more fatal than its omission, which fills asylums with lady patients, terrified by metaphysical translations, and bewildered by religious romances, and who have lost all custom of healthful exertion of body or mind, all love of natural objects, all interest in things most largely influencing the happiness of mankind. All the higher pleasures

* Mental Maladies, p. 235.

of human beings have always been unknown to these patients. Minds so feeble, or so spoiled, are unfit for the ordinary emergencies of a checkered life. Every stronger shock quite discomposes them. These evils have generally taken deep root before the patient's manifest want of reasonable control induces a resort to an asylum; but a large portion of the moral treatment resorted to in asylums consists in the discouragement of the evil habits of mind into which such frivolous and unhappy beings have fallen. Exercise in the open air; customary and general activity; regular hours; a moderate attention to music and other accomplishments, instead of an extravagant devotion of time to such excitements; protection from fanatical exhortations; and the substitution of sensible books for the worthless tracts and volumes with which their well-meaning friends have generally loaded their boxes, and which are thenceforth locked up as so much mental poison, contribute largely to the patient's advance towards rationality. The same kind of care might, in many cases, have preserved the mind from derangement; but the attention of parents and teachers is seldom directed to the important object of the prevention of insanity."*

These and many others that might be mentioned, are undoubtedly predisposing causes of insanity in women. Asks Esquirol, —

"Are not the extreme susceptibility and sedentary life of women, their peculiarities even, the predisposing cause of this malady? The numerous passions which among them are so active; religion, which is a veritable passion with many when love does not exclusively occupy their heart and mind, jealousy, fear, do not these act more energetically on the minds of women than men? As, said Zimmerman, 'insanity comes often to girls from love, to women from jealousy, while from pride to men.' Moreover," continues

* Treatment of the Insane, p. 160.

Esquirol, "women yield to the causes of insanity proper to the sex; physical causes acting more frequently upon them than upon men. Are not women under the control of influences to which men are strangers; such as menstruation, pregnancy, confinement, and nursing?" *

That healthful though continued mental excitement may prevent the tædium vitæ which over-indulgence in the dissipations of society so often brings to women is no paradox, and we should, therefore, have no reason for wonder, if there had in reality been " a decrease of cases of insanity occurring in women since the present war commenced, from the various charitable and benevolent operations which have so largely excited their sympathies and received their support," although, upon the other hand, there would seem to have been at least a counterbalancing number of shocks from sudden bereavement and fright.

That the predisposing or proximate causes, whether moral, mental, or not, — and the physical or ultimate causes rarely act alone, — is no proof of the non-existence of either. They unite and become complicated in many cases where they produce insanity. A fright occasions the suppression of the menses, and this becomes the cause of mania, which ceases with the return of the menstrual evacuation. A woman during her confinement experiences a severe disappointment; the lochia are suppressed, and an eruption of mania takes place. We may with truth affirm that

---

* Mental Maladies, p. 211.

insanity in women rarely takes place without the concurrence of both physical and moral causes.*

It is well known that much of the insanity of women has been attributed, both in asylum reports and elsewhere, to previous general ill health, as owing, in some instances, to the effects of climate, hard work, etc. Upon this point I will subjoin a few remarks that have been communicated to me by my colleague, Dr. Patterson, of the Iowa Asylum.

"It will be seen that among the assigned causes, 'ill health' of various kinds is most prominent. It will seem strange that among the rural population of Iowa, away from the excitements, temptations, excesses, and poverty of large cities, alike remote from the malarious fevers of the South, and the pinching cold of the North, while quietly engaged in the peaceful pursuits of agriculture, any considerable number of our people should ever become insane. And yet such is the fact. Many of them, especially the wives and daughters of farmers, become insane. Probably three fourths of the adult people of Iowa are connected with agricultural pursuits.

"*A vast majority of all cases of insanity arise from causes and circumstances which depress or exhaust the nervous power.* Grief, domestic unhappiness, disappointed affection, the puerperal state, perplexities in business, all tend to depress, and, if long continued, to exhaust the vital force, and are therefore prolific causes of insanity.

"The farmers of Iowa have not yet learned how to live comfortably. Their dwellings are badly constructed, often in low, damp, poorly-drained locations, with either no ventilation, or too much. They are badly warmed by direct radiation of heated iron, so that the process of partial roasting and freezing is at once experienced by the same person

---

* Mental Maladies, p. 382.

Their surroundings are too often unpropitious, their physical comforts and social enjoyments too much neglected. In inclement seasons, amid exposures to cold and rain, their bodies probably receive less care and protection than those of any other class. With abundant supplies at command, their diet is too limited in variety, often unskilfully prepared, and the whole science of gastronomy set at nought. The laboratory, in which are manufactured the life blood and the vital forces, is too often lumbered with ill-assorted, indigestible, badly-cooked food.

"The wives and daughters of farmers, during inclement seasons, have fewer comforts connected with out of doors life, and less adequate protection from cold and humid air, than the women who live in our towns and cities, and it is probable, taking prairie farm life, with all of its surroundings, as it exists in Iowa, that the average standard of the vital force in those who live upon farms, is below that of those who live in the towns and cities. It must not, however, be inferred from these suggestions that the noble and pleasing pursuits of agriculture favor the production of insanity. The errors of living, and the discomforts alluded to, are not necessarily connected with, and certainly not limited to farm life.

"Much of our insanity results from our ignorance or disregard of the laws of animal life. Much of it might be avoided by the exercise of proper care and good judgment in forming alliances, and in the care of our bodies, which are so 'fearfully and wonderfully made;' by ruling the passions and appetites; by lives of prudence; by moderating the extravagant expectations of this life; by using innocent recreations and the bounties of a kind Providence as not abusing them; by regular hours and favoring circumstances for refreshing sleep; by well-regulated households; by an abiding religious faith, and *by the avoidance of those indulgences and habits of life which favor a deterioration of the blood, depress and exhaust the nervous power, and break down the defences which Nature has set up for our protection.*"

There can be no doubt that influences, such as have been above described, do, in many instances, exert a powerful influence upon the nervous system in women, especially if accompanied by disturbance of the pelvic organs, which, indeed, they are so likely to occasion.

The point to which we have now so naturally been brought, — the physical causes of insanity peculiar to women, and their preponderance and efficiency as compared with those of the male sex, — is one that is allowed by many writers, but by most of them is either forgotten or practically contradicted in treatment. Thus Tuke, in his analysis of physical causes, in both male and female, upon a basis of many thousands of cases, places first intemperance, and next epilepsy and disorders more or less connected with the uterus, considering these last as equally productive of insanity, and far more frequently so than all other diseases, or vicious indulgences, or affections of the head and spine, whether idiopathic or traumatic.* A most important allowance has here been made, when it is recollected that of the causes above enumerated, a large proportion of the intemperance of women initiates in or is kept up by alcoholic stimulants, for the purpose of relieving functional or organic uterine disease; that a large proportion of the epilepsy

* Loc. cit., p. 258.

in women is of uterine causation, and that a large proportion of the vicious indulgences of women, especially those of self-abuse, are dependent upon uterine or other local irritation, and so the effect of disease.

I shall present another admission to the same effect from the same author, as it more than corroborates the conclusions to which we shall eventually be brought. He says, —

"When we reflect on the very large number of cases of insanity more or less connected with functional or organic disease of the uterus, and remember that among barbarous nations these disorders are unquestionably of less frequent occurrence than in civilized society, we shall not fail to recognize in this difference one reason why more mental disease might be looked for in the one condition than in the other. Parturition itself, according to the general testimony of travellers, interferes much less, and for a shorter period, with the healthy action of the body and mind among savage nations than among the luxurious daughters of artificial life." *

Dr. Bucknill says, —

"There can be no doubt that uterine disorders constitute one of the most frequent remote causes of insanity with which we are acquainted. If, therefore, the physician can ascertain that his patient has suffered, or is suffering from gastric, hepatic, intestinal, or uterine disease, he will have discovered a well-known and frequent cause, the existence of which must be allowed to exercise its due influence in the diagnosis."

"Disordered states of the abdominal viscera," he again remarks, "are of such frequent occurrence, that the veteran

* Loc. cit., p. 57.

Jacobi and some other physicians of eminence, have believed that they altogether account for the causation of mental disease. We are far from being able to concur in this narrow view of the etiology of insanity; but no physician of much experience in this department of medical science will be likely to deny, that disordered states of the stomach, the intestines, and the liver, frequently constitute the remote causes of cerebral disease."*

It will be remembered that many of the disordered states of the stomach, the intestines, and the liver in women are directly dependent upon uterine derangement, being either caused or kept up by this.

We are told by another writer, that —

"The functions peculiar to the female sex, and the natural sensitiveness of the nervous system in the latter, render them very liable to disturbance of the mind when those functions are irregularly performed. From the commencement of puberty to the approach of old age, this source of disordered nervous and mental action exists, and in every case of insanity occurring in females, the possibility of some bodily functional derangement existing simultaneously with, and, perhaps, operating as the exciting cause of, the mental affection, should never be forgotten. Amenorrhœa, dysmenorrhœa, menorrhagia, pregnancy, miscarriages, parturition, the puerperal state, lactation, the cessation of the menstrual function, are each occasionally productive of mental disorder, which can only be cured by attention to the exciting cause. This consequence of such ailments is naturally rendered much more probable when moral disturbing causes are also in action." †

The frequent coincidence of an uterine crisis or of uterine disease with insanity in woman, must be

---

* Loc. cit., p. 280.
† Robinson: Physical Causes of Mental Disorders, p. 115.

allowed. It has been claimed, however, that this coincidence is one only of time and not of character, that there exists between them no relation of cause and effect. By no one has this assertion been made more succinctly or more emphatically than by the present superintendent of the hospital at Northampton, and late Professor of Psychological Medicine in Berkshire Medical College, Dr. Pliny Earle, whom I therefore quote. He says,—

> "It is well known by persons who have much experience in insanity, that in females there is no constant relationship between the pathological mental condition and the mensual exudation. Some women become insane, continue so for months, and recover, without any interruption of the regularity of their monthly periods. In some the mental disorder precedes, while in others it follows the suppression of the menses. When these have been suppressed, either before or after the invasion of insanity, they may return without having any curative effect upon the mental disease. Some patients recover soon after the reappearance of them, others before their reappearance. When the menses continue regularly through the progress of insanity, in some cases there is an exacerbation of the physical and psychical excitement at the periods, but in others, and I believe it may be said the majority, no such exaltation occurs."*

The above statement, which was made only as part of an argument against the then too frequent resort to bleeding at asylums, might be fully allowed, and yet in no way materially affect the truth of the theory, that upon the state of the uterine system often depends

---

* American Journal of Insanity, x. 398.

the cerebral or mental integrity of women. The occurrence or non-occurrence of the menses, their existence, deficiency, or excess, are but a single one of the many important questions involving a reflex influence by the uterus or ovaries. But even here it will be seen that there is room in every case for much careful investigation, regarding the frequency of the discharge and its coincidence with the usual standard, as to time of appearance, its duration and the length of the interval; its abundance or deficiency; its consistence as to fluidity, and the presence or not of clots, and its odor; its bland or irritating character; its accompaniment or not by pain as a precedent, accompaniment, or consequent; its alternation, connection, or supplantation with or by a leucorrhœal discharge; all these are points without due attention to which all expressions of doubt or discredit are plainly unfounded. If it be, as I have suggested, that the depurative character of the catamenia as eliminating, alternately or in conjunction with the lungs, any excess of carbon from the system, is here efficiently in action, we cannot by a stroke of the pen destroy its influence upon the causation of insanity.

Allowing the coincidence of mental and uterine disturbance, and that the two are in some way connected, it may be asserted that the latter is the consequence of the former, rather than its cause. Thus

Dr. Kellogg points out that the influence of strong mental emotion upon the menstrual secretion is very marked. There are few women of intelligence who have not noticed the fact, and this influence is particularly marked in any of the usual disorders of menstruation. Menorrhagia is almost invariably aggravated by powerful mental emotions. Some forms of dysmenorrhœa are not only caused, but rendered more painful, by mental or moral disturbance.* "Acute suppression of the menses may arise," says Churchill, "from a bodily or mental shock received either just previous to, or during menstruation;" and he gives, in a note, the following interesting illustration of this: —

"Almost all the women who are sent up to the Richmond Penitentiary, after being tried at the Recorder's Court, labor under suppression of the menses, in consequence of the mental agitation and distress they have undergone." †

The frequent occurrence of this result, I am ready to freely allow; but it is no proof that the converse may not more frequently obtain. The twofold possibility of action and reaction is only additional evidence that the sympathy, which is so constantly to be observed between the womb and the stomach or the breasts, also exists, and to a marked degree, between the womb and the brain. This interchange of reflex effect, when admitted, tends to throw light upon the

* Am. Journal of Insanity, Apr. 1856, vol. xii. p. 315.
† Diseases of Women, p. 155.

paradox that had puzzled Dr. Earle, who apparently could not understand how functional derangement or functional crisis could in one instance exist as effect and in another as cause. The coincidence at the same time of moral influences, differing or identical, would tend still further to complicate the question, which is, however, usually easily enough solved by recollecting that more than one derangement or lesion may at one time be present in a single organ.

It will be noticed, moreover, as Dr. Brown-Séquard has claimed for the epileptic aura, when originating from an otherwise healthy womb,* that the irritation, though propagated from that organ, may result from an abnormal change in the quality of the blood within its vessels, or of its secretions other than periodical.

Upon these points, as they are all of great practical importance, I shall add a few words from Dr. Bucknill. It will be seen that in more than one connection he clearly mistakes an effect for the cause, and the cause for its effect. He says, —

"There can be no doubt that the sexual instinct is not unfrequently thrown into a state of extreme excitement by pathological changes taking place in the nervous system. This painful form of disease not unfrequently presents itself during the semi-pathological changes of old age. Those who have been distinguished, during a long life, for prudence and propriety in their relations with the other sex, when, from old age, they have one foot in the grave, are sometimes seen to throw off all restraint, and to rush into the most

---

* Medical Times and Gazette, March, 1863.

reckless and disgusting libertinism. Whether or not this change of manners is accompanied by diseased processes in the brain, we have not yet been able to ascertain by observation. This, however, seems highly probable, since we have seen nymphomania end fatally in young women; and in these cases, in addition to false corpora lutea, we have found great cerebral congestion.* Excitement of the sexual functions may depend upon spinal irritation alone, the lascivious ideas being secondary results, just as ideas of food are the results and not the causes of hunger. Nymphomania, as an example of monomania, is, therefore, liable to the objection that it may be a spinal or cerebro-spinal affection, and independent of that part of the brain which is the organ of the mental [functions]." †

The same author, in another connection, again refers to the matter just now under consideration, which is but one of the many and as yet but imperfectly discussed peculiarities I might mention of insane women. He says, —

"Every medical man has observed the extraordinary amount of obscenity in thought and language which breaks forth from the most modest and well-nurtured woman under the influence of puerperal mania; and although it may be courteous and politic to join in the wonder of those around, that such impurities could ever enter such a mind, and while he repudiates Pope's slander, that 'every woman is at heart a rake,' he will nevertheless acknowledge that religious and moral principles alone give strength to the female mind; and that, when these are weakened or removed by disease, the subterranean fires become active, and the crater gives forth smoke and flame." ‡

---

* Dr. Bucknill forgets that the corpora lutea of menstruation, the cicatrices of ovulation without impregnation, are a normal occurrence, and that nymphomania, however extreme, may result from the pruritus reflexly produced by uterine disease, as for instance carcinoma.

† Loc. cit., p. 321. ‡ Ibid., p. 273.

Esquirol tells us that women in a state of demonomania experience a thousand peculiar sensations.

"They believe they are transported to the midnight assemblies of wizards, where they are witnesses of the strangest extravagances. They have intimate communications with the devil or his subordinates, after which, a collapse bringing an end to the attack, they find themselves again in the same place from whence they believed they had been taken. Who does not see in this the last stage of what, perhaps, commences with hysteria? Amidst the obscenities of these meetings, which we shall be cautious about describing, who does not recognize the turpitude of an imagination polluted by the vilest, most obscene, and disgusting debauchery? Who does not recognize a description of the most extravagant, shameful, and ribald dreams? The frequent ecstasies which take place in nervous affections partake of a sublime and contemplative character, if, during its waking hours, the soul is elevated to the contemplation of noble and divine objects. They are erotic, if the mind and heart lull themselves in reveries of love. They are obscene, if when awake one indulges in lascivious thoughts, and if the uterus, irritated and excited, gives place to illusions which are regarded as diabolical practices."*

Some psychologists have attempted to develop the hints given above, by separating from hysteria what they have termed hystero-mania, this being described as "a true mania developed upon a state of hysteria." †
In practice, however, it will be found very difficult to draw the border line.

The fact just before alluded to has not escaped the notice of observers outside of our own profession.

---

* Mental Maladies, p. 245.
† American Journal of Insanity, October, 1860, p. 120.

"It is not all persons," laments Archbishop Sharp, "that do complain of these wicked and blasphemous thoughts and other extravagant fancies, nor all good persons that are thus haunted, but chiefly those that are of a melancholy constitution, or those of the devout sex; women are more thus affected than the other sex. It concerns, therefore, all these persons to look after their bodies, for upon the cure and health of them the cure and health of the mind doth, in a manner, all in all depend."*

Brierre de Boismont very sensibly remarks, —

"It would be very surprising, if with sensations different to those which are experienced by persons in health, the invalid should continue to reason the same as such persons do; it is true, indeed, that the reason would be perverted and strange." †

He elsewhere, in alluding to the fact that erotic hallucinations are far more common in women than in men, endeavors to explain this difference by the greater facility man possesses for gratifying his desires.‡ He should have added to this, that it is more especially owing to the greater and more constant predominance in women of the sexual system.

There is an old proverb that women advanced in life become either angels or devils. The change referred to is owing to the effect upon them of the conditions occurring at the grand climacteric, as effective for good or evil, alike as regards mental, moral, or physical health, as is the establishment of puberty.

Attempts at explanation of these phenomena have

---
* Casuistical Sermons, vol. iii., London, 1716.
† Work on Hallucinations, p. 367.   ‡ Ibid., p. 313.

been made upon other grounds, but upon examination it is found that the difference is one of words rather than of ideas. Thus Bucknill would lay it down as a general rule that in pure dementia, the sexual instinct is greatly weakened or destroyed. He says, —

"This will be found to be the case even in instances where indecent conduct is observable, for such conduct would seem to arise, not from activity of the instinct, but from the loss of modesty, and from inability to appreciate the rules of decorum. In those cases of senile insanity which are attended by lascivious conduct, the form of mental disease more nearly approaches that of mania than that of dementia. There is a mixture of the two states, but the maniacal element preponderates." *

It would seem that there was here present a bias to erotic ideas, without their becoming efficient in act through exertion of the will, just as we frequently see in general practice, where from ovarian, uterine, vaginal, or vulval irritation, the most lascivious dreams and day-dreams may occur, being confessed to upon inquiry; and yet the patient, though restrained by no apparent check, evinces no symptoms of nymphomania, just as a patient may be homicidal without giving sign of what is passing in her mind, or may breathe threatenings and slaughter, though in act perfectly harmless.

There has still another explanation been offered; only occasionally, however, possible of correct application. It is thus stated by Esquirol, who says

* Loc. cit., p. 291.

that women of hysterical tendencies have sometimes seen the devil under the form of a handsome and well-made young man. Doubtless libertines, abusing the weakness of such invalids, may thus have borrowed from the devil his form and power.*

But it is not women alone who are here in danger. The erotic fancies of the insane may well be looked for in some of the trials for bastardy, rape, and adultery that are brought before courts of law. These are no groundless fears. There are many erotic patients who are convinced that they have had intimate relations with men to whom they have scarcely ever addressed a word, but by whom their imagination has been fired. A case to the point is familiar to most psychologists. It is that of a lady who attended the botanical course of a celebrated French professor. After a few lectures she persuaded herself that she was pregnant by this gentleman, advanced though he was in life, and to whom she had never spoken. Nothing dissuaded her from the belief. The menses were suppressed. She became emaciated and lost her appetite. She spent the eighth month in preparing child-bed linen. The ninth and tenth months were passed without confinement. She thought that the reason of this was that there were no labor pains present, so she stood for a long time upon her naked feet in order to provoke them. She

---

* Esquirol, loc. cit., p. 246.

thought that she heard the professor exhorting her to patience, and encouraging her to support the throes favorable to parturition. In other respects she was perfectly rational.*

Brierre de Boismont says, —

"While supposed intercourse with demons is less common than formerly, the hallucinations generally assume the form of an angel, or of men gifted with all the charms which the imagination can bestow upon them. They frequently refer to the head of the asylum." †

We have thus far been speaking, it is true, more particularly of a single class of cases of mental derangement, those attended with peculiar delusions, distressing to the last degree to all the friends of the patient. The remarks are equally applicable to many other forms of insanity, but here their special causation is often and clearly enough to be distinguished. Esquirol says, —

"Irritations, pains, and lesions of the organs of generation are, in some women more particularly, the frequent cause of illusions. They have sometimes, indeed, caused

---

* Esquirol, loc. cit., p. 246.

† Hallucinations, p. 122. The last sentence of this quotation is not uninteresting in connection with some comments made by my colleague, Dr. Van Deusen, upon the communication made by myself to the American Medical Association at the previous meeting. He says, in a letter dated June 28th, 1864, "I was not before aware of the risks and difficulties experienced in making the examinations referred to. I was not aware that any superintendent had been charged with any of the improprieties intimated; that there had been any legal examination, or anything of the kind, to suggest as a parallel the Beale case, or any occurrence in this country or elsewhere to call for the appointment of an advisory medical board, upon that ground." The quotations from the learned authorities whom I have cited, prove the possibility of the charge, and of its actual occurrence, and at least one case in this country has come to my own knowledge.

the insane to mutilate themselves. Erotic female monomaniacs experience all the phenomena of a union of the sexes. They think themselves in the arms of a lover or ravisher. Cancers and ulcers of the uterus are not uncommon among them. The hysterical insane are disposed to attribute to enemies, to the jealous, and to the devil, the constriction of the throat which suffocates them. The flying pains which they experience in the limbs and viscera, give rise to the most painful illusions." *

Contrary to my general intention, I will present, from the same unexceptionable authority, a few cases of this character, plainly illustrating, as they do, the physical cause of the mental disturbance.

A. D. first menstruated at fourteen. The discharge was always scanty and irregular, and permanently ceased at thirty. She was disappointed in love at this time, and became melancholic. Subsequently there occurred the sensation of painful constriction of the throat, and she was constantly rolling up the skin of the neck with her fingers, and crowding it beneath the sternum. There was considerable tension of the abdomen, and this she attributed to the devil having extended a cord from the sternum to the pubes, and another around her neck, upon which he drew, endeavoring to strangle her.

In the notes of the autopsy it is merely mentioned that the abdominal viscera were found agglutinated by an old peritonitis; no examination of the pelvic viscera seeming to have been made.†

* Loc. cit., p. 115. † Esquirol, loc. cit., p. 239.

M., aged forty-nine, was first unwell at fifteen. The menses ceased at forty. From this period she commenced to have headache, and gradually became insane. The abdomen was hard and voluminous, and the patient had constantly her hand upon it. She stated that she had in her uterus an evil spirit in the form of a serpent, which left her neither by day nor by night, and that her organs of generation were not like those of other women, although apparently normal.*

L. was a laundress, and had always been very devout. The menses commenced at fifteen. She married at seventeen, and became the mother of fifteen children. At forty-six the menses became very irregular, but did not cease until fifty-two, her insanity commencing during this interval. She suffered constantly from uterine pains, and alleged that the devil had been her husband for a million years, and that he was the father of her children; that her body was a sack made of the devil's skin, and filled with serpents, toads, and other unclean creatures.†

A woman, who had been subject to dysmenorrhœa, became the mother of an illegitimate child. She afterwards experienced gastro-intestinal disturbances, and, as so often occurs, became a bigot. At the final cessation of the catamenia she became maniacal, and entered an asylum. She now believed that Pontius

* Ibid., p. 240.   † Ibid., p. 242.

Pilate had been the father of her child, and that he had taken up permanent residence in her bowels, where also the popes held frequent council, being visited at times by the prophets and evangelists, and all the illustrious personages of the Testaments.

At the autopsy, the pelvic viscera were found closely united by peritonitic adhesions, but were not properly examined.

Another patient, in whom the same lesion was discovered after death, believed that she had several devils in her belly, who were constantly tempting her to destroy herself.

A female monomaniac, previously affected with hysteria, was convinced that serpents and other animals, and even the devil, introduced themselves into her body through the genital organs.

Another patient, in confinement at an asylum, imagined that she had in her bowels a regiment of soldiers, and that she could feel them fighting and struggling with each other. When the pains were exacerbated she became excited, crying out that the soldiers were giving blows to each other with their weapons, and at the same time were wounding her entrails.*

A woman insisted that she was pregnant by the devil. She died, and her womb was found distended by a mass of hydatids.†

* Esquirol, loc. cit., p. 114. † Ibid., p. 211.

H. did not menstruate until twenty-four years of age, and since then had been subject to headache and colicky pains. At her third and last confinement, she had a difficult labor, which was followed by attacks of syncope. From this period she imagined that the devil had stolen her body, leaving only a phantom.*

"In many cases of monomania," says Ray, "the hallucination is excited and maintained by impressions propagated by diseased parts, the presence of which has been revealed by dissection after death." †

Such instances as these are not uncommon. I have myself seen several of them, but shall not narrate them at the present time, as I wish here to draw my data from superintendents themselves, whose authority and whose admissions cannot be gainsaid. A case almost identical with that last given, and clearly dependent upon uterine disease, was sent to the Somerville Asylum, by my direction, during the last year.

Instances of supposed pregnancy by the devil, or criminal intercourse with his majesty, are probably more common than was thought by Brierre de Boismont. A case has been referred to by many writers, where exorcism was successfully practised by St. Bernard. A precisely similar instance came into my own hands several years since, in which an equally beneficial result was produced with the aid of a priest.

* Ibid., p. 241.   † Medical Jurisprudence of Insanity, p. 159.

In certain instances, it would not be surprising if such delusions were entertained by superstitious minds, otherwise perfectly sound. I refer to the not uncommon cases of the so-called pseudo-cyesis or spurious pregnancy, to which attention has so forcibly been called by Simpson.* In this affection, as is well known, there are present many of the signs of pregnancy, enlargement of the abdomen and breasts, arrest of the menstrual function, sympathetic derangement of the stomach, and oftentimes a spasmodic and irregularly clonic contraction of the recti and other muscles of the abdomen, closely resembling in their effect the movements of a fœtus in utero. It is sometimes as difficult in these instances to persuade the patient herself that she is not pregnant, as it is her friends; and if she is conscious of never having had intercourse with man, she readily imagines that it has been an immaculate or otherwise supernatural conception.

But I must defer to another occasion my comments upon this and similar points in utero-mental pathology, though the explanations that I would offer are, I believe, in their application original and of very practical importance.

There are one or two matters, however, of such medico-legal bearing that I should do wrong to omit

* Obstetric Works, Scotch Ed., vol. i. p. 300; Clinical Lectures on Diseases of Women, p. 276.

them. Believing as I do that obstetric jurisprudence has been one of the most neglected, as it is one of the most important, of the branches of State medicine, I desire, by the investigation of these questions relating to insanity in women, to contribute somewhat to its advance, as I have previously endeavored to do in my treatise upon criminal abortion.*

The first point to which I shall allude may seem a trivial one. It is that of a morbid and extreme fondness for pets, among women living solitary or secluded lives, and is most commonly brought out in courts during the decision of civil cases. In one suit, for instance, that is on record, it was charged that the testatrix was insane, because she kept fourteen dogs of both sexes, with their kennels, in her drawing-room; two of them slept in her chamber, and one of them, which was blind, in the same bed with her;† another lady kept her sitting-room filled with monkeys, to the great annoyance of her visitors; others have not been happy unless surrounded by parrots, or their room converted into aviaries for all kinds of birds. In one celebrated case, that of Mrs. Cummings, there was exhibited a propensity for cats, which were provided with their meals at table at regular hours, and were furnished with napkins.‡

---

* Criminal Abortion in America: Philadelphia, Lippincott & Co., 1860. Criminal Abortion; its Nature, its Evidence, and its Laws: Boston, Little, Brown & Co., 1869.

† Yglesias *v.* Dyke, Prerog. Court, 1852.

‡ Taylor, Medical Jurisprudence, p. 658. See also Dryden *v.* Fryer, Q. B., Dec. 1850; Journal of Psychological Medicine, 1851, p. 285.

"This propensity for animals proves nothing in relation to the existence of insanity," says Taylor, "unless there is good evidence of mental aberration." On the other hand, it has often been illustrative of decided monomania, and I believe is generally dependent upon ovarian or uterine irritation.

Within a few years a class of cases has made its appearance, exceedingly embarrassing to the medical jurist. These cases are not uncommon. Their description I shall now submit, from Dr. Ray.

"The woman, after preparing for a union to which her head and heart had apparently fully consented, and going through the marriage ceremony with the utmost propriety, manifesting all the while nothing unusual in her deportment, immediately after imbibes an insuperable aversion towards her husband, shuns his company, and perhaps refuses to live with him. In some of the cases, other singularities of conduct soon appear, one after another, till at last the woman becomes a subject of unequivocal insanity. In others, however, this strong repugnance towards the husband continues to be the principal, if not the only, symptom of mental disorder; but so closely do they resemble the former in other respects, that we can have no hesitation in regarding them as merely varieties of the same affection. The pathological character of these cases seems to be sufficiently obvious. From some cause or other, the patient has been affected with a cerebral irritation, not sufficient to disturb the mental manifestations, and which, under favorable circumstances, might have entirely disappeared. In this condition, marriage, with the crowd of new thoughts and feelings by which it is preceded, operates as a powerfully exciting cause, and under its influence the pathological affection is completely developed. It is not strange, certainly, that marriage should occasionally find a female brain in this morbid condition; nor that, in case of such a conjunction, the result here mentioned should follow. The legal relations of these cases are not so satisfactorily settled. In some of them, a close scrutiny of the conduct and condition previous to marriage may detect indubitable signs of insanity; while in others no such signs can be discovered, though subsequently the mental disorder may have become no less obvious. Now, are we prepared to make a distinction between them? To grant divorce in one class and refuse it in the other? This, no doubt, would be highly convenient, but we are not sure that it would be strictly just. While we see not how legal relief can be withheld in the former class, yet in regard to the latter, we recoil from the idea of depriving a woman of her protection and support at the very moment when the severest of earthly calamities has overtaken her, merely on the strength of what we may call a pathological abstraction."*

To the explanation above given by Dr. Ray, I will add two others, which seem to have escaped his notice. In some of these cases the woman gets her first intimation, at or soon after the time of marriage, that her husband has previously had to do with others of her sex, and, as in more than one instance that has come to my knowledge, she shows her disappointment and her disgust accordingly. In other cases, as is well known, the conjugal approach is attended with excessive pain. This effect, normal with the first coitus, at times becomes persistent and a veritable disease; exhibiting itself either in the hyperæsthesia of the vulva, which has been termed vaginismus by Dr.

---

* Medical Jurisprudence of Insanity, p. 240.

Marion Sims, or in an extreme sensibility to touch on the part of the uterus itself. Of both these affections I have seen many cases; in one of the former, the husband had applied for a divorce on the ground that his wife is an hermaphrodite, whereas she is in reality perfectly formed. In one of the latter, the patient having been sent to me by Dr. Walker, of the City Lunatic Hospital at South Boston, on the ground that insanity was threatened, the husband, he said, had been driven to adultery by the practical uselessness, for marital purposes, of his wife.

I have spoken of obscenity and lascivious conduct in women, as the result of disease. There is no doubt that the same explanation is applicable to a large proportion of the cases of so-called self-abuse, which are not uncommon, and are frequently carried to an insane extreme; though insanity, as its consequence, is less frequently occasioned than in men, from the absence of a corresponding exhaustive discharge. So far from being considered and treated as a vice, or from being considered and treated only by moral means, these cases should very frequently be conducted as any others of physical disease. The irritation of ascarides, hæmorrhoids, or mere constipation, of morbid states of the catamenia, of the urine, or of the vaginal secretions, or lesions of the organs themselves, may each and all of them rest at the foundation of the habit, as efficient causes, without whose removal no cure can be hoped for or obtained.*

There are other cases, to a still greater degree involving the mental integrity and the moral responsibility of women. Cases of intemperance, habitual or periodical, of mendacity, of theft, of jealousy, of homicide. Had I not already trespassed so largely upon the patience of the Association, I would present at this time the valuable material I have in my possession relating to what I consider should be the true legal responsibilities of woman, their extent, and whether they should be confined, either as regards their character, or the time of their occurrence, to any particular periods or epochs of her life. This subject has not escaped the observation of Michelet,† and in reference to its relations with pregnancy has attracted the attention of Sedgwick ‡ and others.§ I believe not only that the execution of pregnant women should be stayed for the sake of the life of the child, examination by a jury of matrons, instead of by skilled medical men, being a farce, whose occurrence at the present day is alike a disgrace to the law and to civilization; but that no pregnant or parturient woman, for a crime committed during her gestation, or shortly after her confinement, should ever be executed at all.

---

* See the Journal of the Gynæcological Society of Boston, August, 1870. p. 100.
† L'Amour, p. 334.
‡ Medical Critic and Psychological Journal, October, 1863, p. 694.
§ American Journal of Insanity, January, 1856, p. 295.

A few words upon this point, based upon sound analogy, I shall extract from the work of a well-known and well-educated veterinary surgeon, and shall incidentally refer to the subject again in the course of this report.

Mayhew says, —

"Some bitches cannot be induced to suckle the pups they have given birth to, and others, though less frequently, will eat their progeny. The disposition to desert or destroy their young seems to prevail among the parentage of this world. In the female of the dog the maternal instinct is most powerful; but under certain conditions of the animal's body, the natural impulse seems to be perverted, and she takes the life she would else have perished to preserve. It is painful, knowing this, to reflect that on his own species man inflicts the highest punishment for an act that possibly may be, in the human being as in brutes, the consequence of a mental excitement accompanying the period of parturition. Women not in distress and otherwise afflicted, rarely indeed are guilty of infanticide; and I have observed annoyance of ill health precede or accompany the like act in animals. If the rabbit be looked at, her alarm seems to change her nature; and the bitch that devours her pups will, upon inquiry, be generally found to have suffered some species of persecution. That the brain is affected there can be no doubt. The unnatural propensity is itself a proof; but the strange appearance and altered looks of the creature sufficiently denote her state. She is not then savage, her ferocity has been gratified, and she seems rather to be afflicted with a remembrance of the acts she was unable to resist. She is the picture of shame; she shrinks away at our approach, and her eye no longer confidently seeks that of her master; her aspect is dejected, but I think more with sorrow than with crime. I would not plead for sin; but what I have beheld in dogs induces me to think that the majority of those who have been hung for infanticide were legally murdered. There is danger in admitting such an opinion; but seeing all animals at certain periods exhibit a certain propensity, it is very doubtful whether the morbid feeling, as exemplified in the human race, is really one that calls for mortal punishment." *

Jörg, of Leipsic, who erred in his estimate of the legal and real value of the human fœtus, as I have elsewhere shown,† has expressed a very sensible opinion upon the responsibility of women during pregnancy and parturition, believing that pregnancy can so disturb the intellectual faculties that the patient becomes unable to control her propensities.‡ Montgomery, on the other hand, one of the most profound and most classical writers of modern medicine, believes that "this doctrine is as abhorrent from truth and nature, as it is calculated to lead to the most serious consequences," § thus indorsing the views of Capuron and Devergie, who considered that such an opinion as I have described "would, by taking away all moral responsibility, be fraught with most disastrous results to society;" ‖ although, as I shall now show, the Irish physician, like many another close observer who does not dare to follow his own data to their legitimate conclusions, most emphatically contradicts himself.

* Dogs: their Management, p. 217.
† Criminal Abortion in America, p. 58.
‡ Die Zurechnungsfähigkeit der Schwangern und Gebarenden.
§ Signs and Symptoms of Pregnancy, p. 39.
‖ Médecine Legale, i. p. 433.

VII. — RATIONALE OF PELVIC CAUSATION OF INSANITY.

As throwing some light upon the theory of the causation of insanity in woman by reflex uterine action, or what Forbes Winslow has called the dynamical sympathies of the reproductive organs,* it may not be amiss if I present a few remarks concerning the nervous derangements of pregnancy, from the author I have just quoted, my friend, the late Dr. Montgomery of Dublin. I have selected the period of pregnancy rather than the puerperal state, concerning the mental disturbances of which we have had so much light from the pens of Dr. Gooch, and more recently Drs. Gundry of the Dayton Asylum, and Simpson of Edinburgh; because pregnancy, in itself considered, is rather a normal and physiological, than a pathological condition, its mental abnormal manifestations being of almost identical character with those attending the catamenial crises and climacteric epochs, lesser or greater, not more frequently evinced than at these times, nor more decidedly, if indeed they are not softened down and palliated by the influence of gestation, as sometimes seems to be the case. Whether this, however, or the converse be true, there can be no doubt that the manifestations to which I

* Journal of Psychological Medicine, April, 1854, p. 474.

would refer are clearly and undoubtedly of sexual origin. Montgomery says, —

"When speaking of the physical changes which the uterine system undergoes in consequence of impregnation, it was remarked that the nerves distributed to the organ and its appendages were augmented in size and number, and having their sensibility exalted,* diffused throughout the system generally an increase of nervous irritability, which, affecting both mind and body, displays itself under a great variety of forms and circumstances, rendering the female much more excitable and more easily affected by external agencies; especially those which suddenly produce strong mental or moral emotions, whether of the exhilarating or depressing kind, as fear, joy, sorrow, anger. The powerful influence of such impressions over the functions and actions of the uterus, in every stage of female life after puberty, is recognized in a multiplicity of circumstances, whether as deranging menstruation, inducing abortion, modifying the energy of parturient action, or affecting the recovery from childbed.† Hence the importance of preventing, as far as possible, pregnant women from being exposed to causes likely to distress, or otherwise strongly impress their minds. Sights of an affecting kind, books, pictures, or theatrical representations, which may deeply excite the imagination, or engage the feelings, are decidedly unsafe, and, in illustration of the dangers which may thence arise, I shall mention one or two instances.

"I was once urgently called to see a lady who had gone to the theatre, when two months pregnant, to witness some grand spectacle, in which armed knights on horseback were to cross a bridge and storm a castle; while doing so, the bridge gave way, and the besiegers were precipitated into the torrent beneath, and some of them much hurt. The

---

* It is not necessary to suppose the uterine nerves augmented, either in size or in number, to account for an exaltation of their sensibility.

† Burrows: Commentaries on Insanity, p. 378; Merriman: Synopsis, etc., pp. 33, 224.

lady was dreadfully terrified, screamed, fainted, and was carried home almost insensible, when it was discovered that she was flooding profusely; under the influence of which, and the previous fright, she soon became alarmingly exhausted. However, by the adoption of proper measures, she was restored and tranquillized; but she miscarried before morning. Another case was that of a lady, who, after passing several years of her life in straitened circumstances, and actively employed, married when no longer very young, and was thereby placed in a position of comparative affluence, which, unfortunately for herself, enabled her to dispense with any further exertion, and to indulge a natural inclination to indolence and sedentary habits. She soon became pregnant, and spent her whole time lying on a sofa at the fireside, or with her feet on the fender, reading novels, eating and drinking heartily, and having a discharge from the bowels perhaps once or twice in the week. Amongst the books which she thus daily devoured, was one containing a highly-wrought description of one of the Maisons de Santé in France, and of its inmates; this affected her strongly, and took great hold on her mind, and she expressed the greatest desire to visit one of the large lunatic asylums in this city, that she might assure herself of the reality of such things as she had been reading of. In this wish she was indulged, as in everything else, whether right or wrong, to which she took a fancy; and the consequence was, that the appearance of the persons she had seen, and their extravagant expressions and gesticulations, continued to haunt her imagination incessantly up to the time of her delivery; on the third day after which she showed symptoms of insanity, which became rapidly confirmed, and continued for many months. During her illness, and after her recovery, she repeatedly told me that from the time of reading the book and visiting the asylum, she felt as if she would certainly become deranged.*

"The irritation of the nervous system is in some most obviously perceived in the change induced in the moral

* Signs and Symptoms of Pregnancy, p. 17.

temperament,* rendering the individual depressed and despondent, or, perhaps, she who was naturally placid and sweet-tempered, becomes peevish, irritable, and capricious to a degree as distressing to herself as it is disagreeable to others; yet over this she has little control, and, therefore, much allowance must be made for such waywardness, which, instead of exciting opposition, resentment, or reproach, should claim our utmost indulgence and commiseration; and our best endeavors to comfort, soothe, and cheer. A lady of rank and very superior acquirements told me," he continues, "that for the first two or three months of her pregnancies, she became so irritable that, to use her own words, she was a perfect nuisance in her house, and was so painfully conscious of it herself, that she would sometimes remain in bed all day, or confine herself to her room, to avoid displaying her irritability to the annoyance of others. This lady has since died of cancer uteri, under the most deplorable circumstances.

"I have known the effect produced to be the reverse of this, and a decided amelioration take place in the temper, as we sometimes also see happen in the exercise of the bodily functions during pregnancy, A gentleman once informed me that, being afflicted with a stepmother naturally more disposed to practise the fortiter in re than to adopt the suaviter in modo, he and all the household had learned, from experience, to hail with joyful anticipations the lady's pregnancy as a period when clouds and storm were immediately exchanged for sunshine and quietness.

"Some suffer most from this irritability depriving them of sleep, night after night, especially if they have not guarded against feverishness by proper attention to the state of the bowels, or sleep in rooms too warm or insufficiently ventilated; and yet it is singular how little they appear to suffer from this loss of rest, seeming really as much recruited by the short snatches of sleep which they obtain as they would, at other times, when enjoying unbroken repose. Others sleep, but suffer even more from painful and distress

---

* Harvey, 4to. edition, p. 593.

ing dreams; while some are liable to annoyance of a totally different kind, being constantly so drowsy, that it is with difficulty they can keep awake, even in company.

"I suppose many have noticed a curious fact connected with the state of mind in pregnant women, when their bodily health is at the same time good, namely, that however depressed or dispirited with gloomy forebodings they may have felt in the early part of their pregnancy, they, in general, gradually resume their natural cheerfulness as gestation advances, and, a short time before labor actually commences, often feel their spirits rise and their bodily activity increase to a degree that they had not enjoyed for months before. I have known instances in which this took place so regularly and distinctly, in successive pregnancies, that the patients were able, from its occurrence, to anticipate and announce the near approach of their labor. This must strike us as a wise and beautiful arrangement by which, on the eve of suffering, the mind rises with a spring to meet the trial with cheerfulness and fortitude, which experience proves so materially to contribute to a happy result.

"Occasionally, however, the depression assumes a more serious aspect, and the woman is constantly under the influence of a settled and gloomy anticipation of evil, sometimes accompanied with that sort of apathetic indifference which makes her careless of every object that ought naturally to awaken an interest in her feelings; a state which we sometimes observe in fever and other severe disorders, in which it is justly considered a most unfavorable symptom. When this occurs in pregnancy, it will generally be found accompanied by very evident derangements in bodily health; a dull heaviness, or aching of the head, a loaded tongue with bitter taste in the mouth, constant nausea, costiveness, and a foul state of the alvine discharges, with not unfrequently a bilious tinge in the skin, and other symptoms indicating hepatic derangement, together with a quick pulse and a dry, hot skin, constitute the group of symptoms likely to be present, and which urgently demand attention for their removal before the time of labor, otherwise serious consequences are to be apprehended. Sometimes this state appears to depend on some peculiar condition of the brain, the nature of which we probably cannot appreciate, and which our treatment will but too often fail to correct; in one strongly-marked instance of this kind, which was some time ago under my care, the lady became maniacal on the fifth day after delivery, and continued deranged for many months."

Reasoning by analogy from such considerations as those we have just been engaged in, we should be led to expect as probable, what experience confirms as certain, that occasionally the cerebral disturbance during pregnancy, which, in most instances, only shows itself in unevenness of spirits, or irritability of manner or temper, amounts in some to absolute disorder in the intellectual faculties, especially in habits naturally very excitable, or where there is an hereditary predisposition. Dr. Prichard says,—

"If we consider the frequent changes or disturbances occurring in the balance of the circulation from the varying and quickly succeeding processes which are carried on in the system during and soon after the periods of pregnancy and childbirth, we shall be at no loss to discover circumstances under which a susceptible constitution is likely to suffer. The conversions, or successive changes in the temporary local determinations of blood, which the constitution under such circumstances sustains and requires, appear sufficiently to account for the morbid susceptibility of the brain." *

"One cannot deny," says Roussel, "that the minds of pregnant women are singularly modified;" † and

---

* Treatise on Insanity, p. 312.   † Système de la Femme, p. 160.

this susceptibility to mental disturbance, on the part of the mother, has been recognized on high authority as giving rise to one species of congenital predisposition to insanity in the offspring. In some, this sensorial agitation may be confined to the more strongly marked forms of hysteria, or only exhibit itself in those unaccountable phantasies called longings, "which," says Dr. Burrows, "are decided perversions or aberrations of the judgment, though perhaps the simplest modifications of intellectual derangement,"* but in others it is truly, and even violently, maniacal. "I have, on one occasion," says Montgomery, "noticed a case where mania occurred in eight successive pregnancies, and another in which the woman was three times similarly affected soon after conception, and remained deranged until within a short time of her labor, when she became sane, and continued so until the recurrence of pregnancy."† "Some," again remarks the author last quoted, "are insane in every pregnancy or lying-in, others, only occasionally."‡ Marc, writing on the same subject, says, "I recall a patient in Esquirol's Asylum, in whose case the commencement of each pregnancy was characterized by an attack of transient insanity."§ Goubelly relates a case of an opposite kind, in which the lady was of sound mind only during her

---

* Commentaries on Insanity, p. 147. † Dublin Medical Journal, v. p. 52.
‡ Loc. cit., pp. 364-378.   § Dict. de Sc. Méd., xix. p. 489.

pregnancies, but was then deficient in memory; of which latter defect the following is a remarkable instance: —

"A fright produced by the dangerous situation of her only son when eighteen months old, brought on, in Mrs. Durant, an alarming illness, attended with some singular phenomena, the most singular of which respected her memory. The illness happened in July, when she was advanced six months in a state of pregnancy, and was, when perfectly insensible, delivered of a child. On awaking from her insensibility, which had continued for three days, she imagined it was the month of January. Her mental powers generally were but slightly impaired, and soon regained their former perfection; nor was her memory affected, except as regarded the preceding six months. Of that time she had forgotten all the events: some accidental circumstance might afterwards occasionally produce a train of thought, which would bring an event of those six months to her recollection; but several of the most important were never regained, nor could she, to the hour of her death, remember that she had then been pregnant. I have met with a few instances in which the memory was similarly effaced, and under apparently similar circumstances, but for much shorter periods of time." *

It has been asserted that manifestations such as those we have now seen described, whether occurring in pregnancy, at or after childbed, or during any other time of a woman's life, are merely attacks of hysteria, as distinguished from actual insanity, more or less aggravated as these may be. The error of such a supposition has been allowed by more than one psychologist. I have already called attention to the similar error of endeavoring to separate in all cases

* Montgomery, Signs and Symptoms of Pregnancy, pp. 32–37.

from hysteria the so-called hystero-mania. In some cases, however, of hysteria, the mania may be counterfeited. Dr. Bucknill says, —

"The diagnosis between exaggerated hysteria and incomplete primary mania must be made by observing the sex, age, constitution, and character of the patient, which, to the experienced physician, will generally reveal the nature of hysterical attacks, whatever form they may assume. They do sometimes assume the form of mania, with violent general excitement and strongly pronounced moral perversions. These may be looked upon as the proper symptoms of the disease; but hysterical patients have been known to feign delusions and hallucinations, just as they will feign everything else. The hysterical type of the patient, the paroxysmal nature of the excitement, and the contradictions in which she may be detected when closely examined upon the circumstances of her supposed delusions, will rarely fail to detect the comparatively harmless nature of the affection. This will be the more easy, if the effect of remedies appropriate to hysteria can be tried. But hysteria does sometimes pass into real mania, and carry with it some of its own peculiarities. In all the instances in which we have observed this transition, there has been a strong hereditary tendency to insanity. The transition has been marked by an obvious febrile crisis, and by that most important symptom of early mania, loss of sleep. The medical man must, therefore, exercise due caution, in avoiding to pronounce any case to be purely hysterical because it has once been so. If, in a young woman of hysterical temperament, the perverted sentiments and desires, the strange conduct and excited demeanor pass into a febrile stage, accompanied by a rapid pulse, by loss of sleep, and by delusion or hallucination, hysteria has passed into mania. Patients are even met with, in whom periods of hysterical and maniacal excitement alternate; and it is not difficult to distinguish in them the period when the superficial disorder presents itself, and when it yields to the more profound and serious disease." *

With respect to hysteria, we are told by Dr. Montgomery, although in its ordinary or slighter forms, it is not perhaps properly deserving the name of mental disturbance, its more aggravated conditions are so closely allied thereto, that it must be extremely difficult to draw the line of distinction. "Cases of this kind," says Dr. Conolly, "approach near to insanity; and, indeed, a mind subject to the violent agitations incidental to the hysteric constitution cannot be considered as perfectly sane;" † a state of which Sydenham has given so admirable and graphic a description, in which he says, the patients "observe no mean in anything, and are constant only to inconstancy; so unsettled is their mind that they never are at rest." ‡ Montgomery says, —

"Of one fact, at least, my own experience and that of others afford sufficient evidence, that when the aggravated form of hysteria prevails throughout pregnancy, puerperal mania is much to be apprehended.§ I have also observed, in not a few instances, that women who, at other times, have been the subjects of that slight form of mental unsteadiness which goes by the name of extreme nervousness, and is evinced in an unreasonable susceptibility of impressions from slight causes affecting their moral feelings, but without any perceptible lesion of the intellectual faculties, and constituting probably the simplest form of moral insanity, have

---

* Manual of Psychological Medicine, p. 301.
† Cyclopædia of Practical Medicine, ii. p. 563.
‡ Swan's Translation, ed. 1769, p. 414.
§ Burrows, loc. cit., p. 378.

had their state of mind greatly improved during pregnancy; but soon after the termination of that condition, have exhibited, for a time, a greater degree of mental disquiet than was habitual with them, which, however, again settled down into their ordinary state.

"I desire now to observe that, in thus noticing some of the more remarkable phenomena occasionally displayed during pregnancy, it is not intended to imply that such are the usual concomitants of that condition; on the contrary, most of them are to be considered as rare occurrences, some of them remarkably so, and all as exceptions to the general rule; but, for this very reason, deserving of particular notice, as probably connected with a morbid state of the system, either absolutely existing at the time, though perhaps not otherwise clearly appreciable, or about to be developed, as in the case I have already related, where memory of the whole time of pregnancy was a complete void; my object being to point out forcibly, what experience seems to have fully established, that during pregnancy the system is in a state of unusual susceptibility; the activity of both the nervous and circulating systems being at that time greatly exalted, by which the female is rendered much more liable to be injuriously affected, even by ordinary causes, and still more so by any of a more impressive kind." †

The peculiar manifestations which demonstrate this exaltation of the nervous system are of the most varied character. They are familiar to every obstetrician, and to many of them attention has been called by Montgomery. Some women, for instance, are much troubled with frightful dreams whenever they are pregnant. Dr. Lowder used to relate the case of a lady who was obliged to have a nurse sitting at her bedside all night, to watch her countenance while she

* Signs of Pregnancy, p. 41.

slept, and to awaken her as soon as she perceived her exhibiting distress under the influence of her dreamy terrors. Disorder of the alimentary canal, disturbing the already irritated nervous system, is, probably, the most frequent cause of this affection; it may also be induced by irregular or undue circulation of blood in the brain; relief has been obtained by acting upon such a presumption, administering aperients, and abstracting blood by cupping on the nape of the neck.

According to Beccaria, there is a peculiar kind of headache accompanying pregnancy, which he describes as an acute pulsating pain in the occipital region;[*] occupying particularly the part in which Gall places the organ of the instinct of reproduction. "This pain," he says, "is accompanied with giddiness on the least motion of the head, and with difficulty in supporting the light; it comes on suddenly, and, continuing for some time, is succeeded by an inclination to sleep."[†] It is often perceived.

There is another variety of headache, familiar to all who are conversant with the symptoms of sick women, as almost pathognomonic of uterine disease. It is generally attended with a peculiar and almost indescribable sensation of outward pressure at the vertex, and was excellently described, some years since,

---

[*] Annali Universal. de Med., September, 1830; Archives Générales de Médicine, xxiv. p. 443.
[†] Montgomery, loc. cit., p. 284.

by Dr. Tyler, the present Superintendent of the McLean Asylum.*

Strange appetites, moreover, or longings, as they are called, and antipathies, are well known as frequent attendants on pregnancy in many persons; some of whom will long to eat unusual, and even revolting articles, while others, immediately after conception, are seized with an unconquerable aversion to species of food which were previously particularly agreeable to them. Montgomery says, —

"I have seen several well-marked instances of this, and, in particular, one in the case of a lady who assured me that she always knew when she was with child, by feeling a violent antipathy for wine † and tea, which, at other times, she took with pleasure. I had an opportunity of observing the accuracy of this indication, in the successive pregnancies of the lady alluded to. A patient of Dr. Dewees used to consume enormous quantities of chalk when pregnant; and Capuron knew a woman whose principal food was long pepper, which she used to swallow by handfuls; ‡ under the same circumstances, one patient of mine eats quantities of cloves, for the first three or four months; and another indulges with equal freedom in eating dry oatmeal.

"There is a curious and interesting coincidence between such facts as these, and others not unfrequently observed in certain states of uterine disturbance, connected with suppressed or deranged menstruation; especially about the time when that function is first established, when it is not unusual to find girls eat with avidity the most uninviting

---

* New Hampshire Journal of Medicine, November, 1851, p 62. See also the Journal of the Gynæcological Society of Boston, May, 1870, p. 262.
† This particular aversion was expressly noticed by Hippocrates as a sign of pregnancy, "vinum odio habent." De Infecundis, Cap. 6.
‡ Traité des Accouchemens, p. 42.

substances, such as cinders, dry mortar, or clay; and in a case, about which I was some time ago consulted, the young lady used to pick the bog-wood out of the grate and eat it.

"This morbid state of the appetite did not escape the notice of Ben Jonson, who thus alludes to it:—

> 'She can cranch
> A sack of small coal, eat you lime and hair,
> Soap, ashes, loam, and has a dainty spice
> Of the green sickness.' *

"Such caprices of appetite may at first, perhaps, only excite a smile, but experience appears to have sufficiently shown that their indulgence cannot always be permitted without imminent risk of injury to the mother, or child, or both." †

These propensities, in their essence maniacal and in their demonstratious often clearly so, have received special attention from another British observer, ‡ to whom, however, I should hardly refer at this time had not his explanations of the phenomena in question been evidently accepted as valid by a noted psychologist, Dr. Forbes Winslow, from whose interesting though somewhat poetical article upon woman in her psychological relations, I shall accordingly present a few extracts.

"The modifications of the appetite, says Dr. Laycock, necessary in the female of the lower animals, for the proper nutrition and development of the ovum or fœtus, are occasionally reproduced in the pregnant human female as morbid appetites.

"It has been observed by naturalists that birds will eat lime or chalk while laying — obviously that the shell may be

---
* The Magnetic Lady, Act I. Sc. 1.   † Montgomery, pp. 278, 279.
‡ Laycock: Treatise on the Nervous Diseases of Women.

duly formed; for, if hens be deprived of the opportunity of obtaining it, the eggs have only a membranous covering, or an imperfect shell. So, also, female carnivorous animals have the appetite for their natural food more ravenously excited during utero-gestation and lactation, to the same end: namely, that of duly perfecting the nutrition of the young animal. These morbidly excited appetites are known as 'longings' in the pregnant woman, and in the young unmarried woman as pica and bulimia. This change in the appetites has always attracted popular attention, and given rise to much astonishment, but we are now enabled to trace them to their origin. Dr. Laycock observes, that although during pregnancy some good wives 'long' for handsome dresses, furniture, &c., yet these longings are spurious, since the morbid feelings belong exclusively to the appetite for food. Ben Jonson notices these spurious longings, as follows:—

"'*Littlewit.*— O yes, Win: you may long to see as well as to taste, Win: as did the 'pothecary's wife, Win, that longed to see the anatomy, Win. Or the lady, Win, that desired to spit in the great lawyer's mouth, after an eloquent pleading.'—*Bartholomew Fair*, Act III. Sc. 1.

"Ben Jonson, indeed, seems to have had some experience in this form of morbid appetite, for he refers to it again and again in his plays. Thus, in Act I., of that just quoted, he makes the same character say,—

"'Win, long to eat of a pig, in the fair, do you see, in the heart of the fair, not at Pye-corner. Your mother will do anything, sweet Win, to satisfy your longing, you know; pray thee, long presently, and be sick 'o the sudden, good Win,' &c.

"The things desired in this ovarian perversion of the appetite are sometimes very extraordinary, and outrageously absurd. Dr. Laycock quotes Dr. Elliotson as mentioning in his lectures that a patient has longed for raw flesh (the carnivorous appetite), and even for live flesh, so that some have eaten live kittens and rats. Langius, a German writer, tells a story of a woman who lived near Cologne, who had such a cannibalish longing for the flesh of her husband, that she killed him, ate as much of him as she could while fresh, and pickled the remainder. Another longed for a bite out of a baker's arm. More marvellous masticators than the case described in the play of 'The Magnetic Lady,' from which we have already quoted; although Dr. Laycock quotes the case of a German woman who would eat a bonbonnière of charcoal.

"The 'dainty spice of the green-sickness' is known by some pathologists under the term of 'Temper Disease.' It is attended by the impaired digestion and defective assimilation which characterize chlorosis, and by the most extraordinary perversions of temper, very frequently with regard to diet, the patient persisting in a system of starvation, or only taking the most improper food, or that which she can get by stealth. Here, again, we trace a link of the mysterious chain which connects organism together, and can have little doubt that this form of psychological change is due to a morbid action of the reproductive organs, such as occurs occasionally in pregnancy.

"There are other alterations in the mental character of women belonging to this class of perverted instincts, which are of greater importance, because they involve the social and moral relations. The hysterical cunning of the young female is traced by Dr. Laycock to the same ovarian source. Referring to the development of certain instincts in the female at the period of procreation, and when the care of offspring is the great end of life, he compares the artfulness of the lower animals with this hysterical cunning, and attributes it to the influence of the ovaria on the nervous system.*

"He also observes," continues the reviewer, "that astuteness is as much the characteristic of woman as courage is of man, but that these characteristics are not morbidly developed except under given circumstances. It is not until puberty that these peculiar qualities of the constitution of woman are distinctly brought out; and in brutes it is only when the business of reproduction is carried on, that this artfulness is so exalted as to rival the highest attempts of

* Journal of Psychological Medicine, Jan., 1851, p. 31.

human sagacity. The skill they display in the choice of a secret place in which to deposit their eggs or young, and the finesse with which the latter are protected from discovery or injury, are well known to the most inexperienced student of natural history. The lioness, for example, ferocious and powerful as she is, when she fears the retreat in which she has placed her cubs will be discovered, will hide her footmarks, by retracing the ground, or brushing them out with her tail. When the young female suffers from irregular action of the ovaria on the system, the natural astuteness and quickness of perception degenerate into mere artfulness, or monomaniacal cunning; and it is to this morbid influence of the ovaria on the organ of the mind, that Dr. Laycock attributes the extraordinary instances of monomaniacal cunning in females, on record. He observes, on this head, 'Of all animals, woman has the most acute faculties; and when we consider how much these may be exalted by the influence of the reproductive organs, there is not much ground for surprise at the grotesque forms which cunning assumes in the hysterical female, although they have caused much speculation and astonishment. Insane cunning is usually exhibited in attempts at deception, but occasionally in a propensity to steal, or rather to steal slyly. It may be remarked that, when it occurs, it may be as much a symptom of hysteria as any corporeal affection whatever. It is a true monomania, and is most likely to occur in the female who is hysterical from excess of sexual development— *one possessing the utmost modesty of deportment and grace of figure and movement, for the modesty itself springs out of that feminine timidity to which I have just alluded.* Sly stealing, however, is most frequently observed in pregnant women.' The Italics in the above quotation are our own," says Dr. Winslow, "as we wish to direct the reader's special attention to the important principle pointed out by Dr. Laycock. The propensity, in such case, is dependent solely on the excitement of the nervous system by the ovaria; hence it is that when, in consequence of an active condition of those structures, the graces peculiar to the feminine character are peculiarly developed, and gentleness, modesty, and timidity are prominent characteristics, often in those identical cases it is, that there is this morbid excitation of the instinct of artfulness or cunning; and it is these endowments which explain the influence that hysterical girls have upon all that come near them, and which is really astonishing; parents, women, physicians, all yielding to them. It is also the marked excitation of this sexual artfulness, which renders nugatory all the experiments and labors of those mesmerists, whose principal subjects are young females or youths about the age of puberty. Psychologists, practically acquainted with this subject, can place no reliance upon the statements of the hysterical females upon whom mesmerists experiment, however well educated, gentle, good, and truth-loving they may be naturally, and really are in all other matters. Physicians have recorded numerous instances of strange and motiveless deceptions, thefts, and crimes practised by young women, even by ladies of unexceptionable morals, excellent education, and high rank. Fasting women, ecstatica, sly poisoners, pilfering lady-thieves, &c., present examples of this kind; particular instances we need not mention, as they may be found in most works on hysteria, and often occupy a niche in the newspapers. When cunning is combined with a morbid excitation of the propensity to destroy, such as is manifested in the females of brutes, the effect is sometimes dreadful, and is seen in the perpetration of secret murders by wholesale poisoning, or in secret incendiarism; and if other natural instincts be perverted, the objects of woman's warmest and most disinterested affections may perish by her hand. It is a singular fact in natural history, and remarkably illustrative of our views, that parturient domestic animals sometimes suffer from the same morbid condition of the nervous system as the human mother, and they also destroy their offspring. Thus," as we have already had pointed out by Mayhew, "cats, sows, and bitches have been known to eat their litter; cows to butt their calves to death, hens to chase their chickens, &c.

"When cunning is combined with a morbid state of the temper, the misery inflicted upon domestic peace is inexpressible. The ingenuity in malice and falsehood displayed by the patient, is most extraordinary; so extraordinary, indeed, that it is never credited until it is experienced. Cases are by no means infrequent in which the sufferer from this sad derangement is the most intellectual and most amiable of the family; beloved by all, respected, almost worshipped. Hence, when, after numerous struggles to repress them, the propensities, excited into such fearful and almost supernatural activity by the ovarian irritation, burst forth beyond all control, and the pet of the family is seen to be the opposite, morally, in every respect to what she had been, — irreligious, selfish, slanderous, false, malicious, devoid of affection, thievish in a thousand petty ways, bold, may be erotic, self-willed, and quarrelsome; the shock to the family circle and friends is intense; and if the case be not rightly understood, great, and often irreparable mischief is done to correct what seems to be vice, but is really insanity.

"Perhaps in the whole range of psychology there is no subject so deeply interesting as this; for it is in so-called moral insanity that man's spiritual and moral nature is the most awfully and most distressingly subjected to his corporeal frame. It is a disease, undoubtedly, much more frequent in the female sex than in man." *

Dr. Montgomery says, —

"Dr. Harvey mentioned the case of a lady who, whenever she was pregnant, became affected with the most uncontrollable passion for building; this had taken place several times, and always subsided when pregnancy ceased. A marked change in the temper is very commonly observed, so that a woman who was, under ordinary circumstances, extremely mild and sweet-tempered, immediately becomes, when pregnant, irritable and capricious, an effect which in some women attends each recurrence of pregnancy." †

* Journal of Psychological Medicine, January, 1851, pp. 31, 43.
† Loc. cit., p. 278.

These are clearly and distinctly, to the extent to which each of them goes, cases of a monomaniacal character; which character, in itself considered, is not affected by the possibility of the affection in some cases being intermittent, paroxysmal, or periodical, while in others it is chronic and persistent. There are other abnormal manifestations, even of special sense, of whose occurrence abundant evidence can be afforded.

There is a simulation of disease which occasionally accompanies pregnancy, and depends apparently on disturbance of the nervous influence, which sometimes very remarkably affects the functions of some of the organs of the external senses, in which no appreciable organic change can be at the time discovered; and that none such does really take place, seems sufficiently evident from the fact that the affection lasts only during gestation. Thus, instances of temporary amaurosis induced by pregnancy are by no means uncommon.* Dr. Montgomery says, —

"I saw a lady thus affected; she could see certain objects distinctly, as a line drawn on paper; others appeared confused, and some she could hardly discern at all; occasionally she imagined she saw objects which were not present, as a person crossing the room, or flower-pots, or bunches of flowers on her table, when nothing of the sort was there. Salmutius relates a case in which a lady became blind every time she was pregnant, and recovered her sight as soon as

---

* Good: Study of Medicine, iv. p. 247; Cooper: Surgical Dictionary art. Amaurosis.

she lay in.* Beer saw a young Jewess, who at the very beginning of her first three pregnancies, which followed each other quickly, regularly became amaurotic, and continued blind till after delivery; but on the third occasion she did not recover her sight.† Chambon ascribes these affections to plethora; but such an explanation is scarcely consistent with the occurrence of amaurosis from protracted or undue lactation, when the constitution is in a state of great debility and exhaustion; two well marked instances of which I saw in two sisters, who quickly recovered their sight by weaning their children. Dr. Mathews, of Moate, has just informed me of the case of a lady who, when five months pregnant, for the first time sustained total loss of voice, which she recovered at the time of her labor. Gardien notices this part of our subject fully, and mentions a variety of affections which I have not met with.‡ Dr. Bennewitz has detailed the particulars of a case, in which a young woman was, in three successive pregnancies, affected with diabetes mellitus; which, each time, completely ceased on delivery, but again returned when she became pregnant." §

These physical derangements, of reflex and uterine causation, are sometimes extreme. Thus it is not unusual, during the existence of pregnancy, to find the power of one or both of the lower limbs more or less impaired; and, in some few rare instances, they have bcome partially or completely paralytic, and even hemiplegia has been observed. Montgomery says,—

" To what degree the mere enlargement of the uterus is the agent in the production of such a state (by mechanical pressure) seems very doubtful, especially as we sometimes

---

* Cent. III. Obs. 27.
† Lehre von den Augenkrankheiten.
‡ Traité des Accouchemens, i. p. 437, and ii. 76.
§ Osam: Clinical Report for 1823; Edinburgh Medical Journal, xxx. p. 217 Montgomery, loc. cit., p. 47.

find the paralysis affecting the upper extremities;[*] the blood drawn under such circumstances has been observed to present highly inflammatory characters; but whatever measures may be adopted, the affection is never perfectly removed until after delivery, from which it would appear to depend on cerebral disturbance, originating probably in uterine irritation, and referable to the state of pregnancy as its specific cause." [†]

Of course such cases are to be distinguished from those of paralysis occurring during or after labor, in consequence of apoplectic convulsions, or from undue or long-continued pressure upon the pelvic nerves by the fœtal head.

The evidence that I have now presented proves more than that the state of pregnancy is one subject to grave mental and physical derangement, giving rise to serious anxieties, and requiring judicious treatment. It proves, also, that at the foundation of the whole matter lies an excited uterus. The irritation that, during pregnancy, may coexist, as a normal and physiological state, with the usual or improved health, may, in other cases, assuming a pathological type, or in the presence of pathological adjuncts, cause the inception or development of severe disease. In other words, the tendency to reflex derangement, whether of body or mind, usually attending uterine disturbance, but also usually controlled during pregnancy by the vis medicatrix of impregnation, may at times

---

[*] Edinburgh Monthly Journal, xii. p. 492.
[†] Loc. cit., p. 5.

during this period assume its primal sway, and produce effects, under other circumstances naturally to be expected.

If we change the premises, the same result obtains. I have assumed the excited uterus as a natural cause of reflex disease, as is proved by its conduct at times other than pregnancy, and have shown that the diseases of pregnancy are but the special diseases of other times allowed to exhibit themselves here. Let us now shift the scenes of proof, and assuming pregnancy, however occasionally permitted to occur, as the normal condition of the adult woman, and its processes uninterfered with, and as usually presenting themselves to be strictly physiological in their character, we will compare its diseases, physical and mental, with the special affections of women occurring at other times. They are found to be nearly identical in type, in detail, in their general course and result: a similarity of effect argues an identity of cause. Whichever horn of the dilemma is then selected, its point is the same. If an excited uterus causes the derangements of pregnancy, so it does those of other special times and seasons. If an excited uterus causes the latter, it is by the same mechanism and same reflex causation as that by which the former are occasioned.

As to puberty, for instance: I will quote a word from Dr. Ray.

"That the evolution of the sexual functions is very often attended by more or less constitutional disturbance, especially in the female sex, is now a well-established physiological truth. The shock seems to be felt chiefly by the nervous system, which experiences almost every form of irritation, varying in severity from the slightest hysterical symptoms to tetanus, St. Vitus's dance, and epilepsy. And when we bear in mind, also, that general mania is sometimes produced by this great physiological change, it cannot be deemed an extraordinary fact that partial mania, exciting to acts of incendiarism or murder, should be one of its effects." *

Just as puberal mania may thus be produced, so may there occur the first explosion at any other of the periodic crises, of longer or shorter interval, to which we have seen woman is constantly liable. The climacteric invasion of insanity has lately been studied by Dr. Francis Skae, formerly attached to the Royal Asylum at Morningside,† and it is to be hoped that we may soon have memoirs upon each of the other developmental types to which I have already alluded.

I have now shown that both *à priori*, and from the evidence of experts in insanity, there is reason to believe that their sex lies at the foundation, physiologically and pathologically, of much of the mental derangement that occurs in women. I am well aware that the work has been but imperfectly performed. Had space and a fair allowance for the patience of the Association permitted, I should have presented

---

* Medical Jurisprudence of Insanity, p. 200.
† Edinburgh Medical Journal, Feb., 1865, p. 703.

much additional proof that I am, at present, compelled to withhold.

Negative evidence, no matter what its amount or from what quarter afforded, should not, I would respectfully submit, be allowed to weigh against the positive proof that I have afforded; yet the arguments that can alone be brought to disprove my position are strictly and merely negative in their character. It will be sufficient if I refer to merely one or two of them. From an example we may understand its class.

It has been stated by several writers, — I have already quoted Dr. Earle's opinion upon the subject, — that the regular occurrence, absence, or suppression of the catamenia seems in many cases to have made no difference as to the causation, continuance, or cure of insanity in women, and that therefore the uterus and ovaries are proved incapable of exerting any appreciable influence as an agent in the production of the mental disease. The error that is here present is an evident one: it is in considering that in all uterine or ovarian diseases there must be derangement of a single function, that of menstruation, or that the presence and partial or complete performance of this function argues uterine health. Such an argument only proves most lamentable ignorance, even of the most common and simplest of the diseases of women, and of which the youngest medical student of the present day would be ashamed.

Again, it must not be forgotten that the diseases special to women are now recognized to embrace a vast variety of simple and complex lesions, equalling in number, if not excelling, those of any other organ or system of organs in the body. The wise physician of old was not far wrong in his judgment: "What is woman? Disease, says Hippocrates." * The absence of one affection, of whatever class, in any given patient, is no evidence that another may not exist. Am I wrong, then, in advising more careful examinations than are commonly made, even in general practice?

Still further, it has been asserted, that because many insane women make no complaint of pelvic pain, we ought, from that fact, to take for granted the non-existence of uterine disease. This statement would hardly be made were it recollected — for every medical man, however long retired from active practice, must once have known — that even among sane patients cases are not so very uncommon of advanced and decided uterine disease when the only pains present are reflex, and exhibited merely as distant neuralgias of the back, face, breast, or other location. Indeed, I may state that I have seen, in quite a number of instances, the uterus nearly destroyed by malignant disease, without a trace of the lancinating pain that authors have too much insisted upon as necessary, however generally pathognomonic when it does exist,

* Michelet: L'Amour.

and the patient hardly aware of any local discomfort. That such cases do occur in the sane, only strengthens the argument I have elsewhere dwelt upon, quoting Bucknill and other authorities; that while the peculiar tolerance of pain, so often observed in the insane, is now allowed frequently to veil the existence of phthisis and similar forms of organic disease, just as it does of wounds and injuries, so must it be granted that at times there may exist and progress any and every form of uterine and pelvic lesion without its coming to the knowledge of the physician or asylum superintendent, unless he suspect its occurrence, and search therefor.

As a single instance from many that might be given, I append a statement by Dr. Tuke, attached to the Royal Lunatic Asylum at Morningside, near Edinburgh. In presenting to the Edinburgh Obstetrical Society, at its meeting in January, 1865, specimens of fibroid tumor and polypus of the uterus, removed, post-mortem, from a woman who had been in the asylum for twenty years, without ever making complaint of pelvic disturbance, this gentleman remarks, —

"I was not aware of the existence of the tumor until I examined her amongst other patieuts, making a careful investigation into the bodily health of all the old inmates, with the view of discovering diseases which are liable to lie latent in the insane, to an extent hardly to be credited by any but those accustomed to their treatment." *

* Edinburgh Medical Journal, March, 1865, p. 857.

And, finally, I have been told by some gentlemen, that because many women have disease of the uterus, detected during life, without insanity, and by others, that because at autopsies of sane patients, similar disease, undetected during life, because unlooked for, has been discovered; so must it therefore be admitted, that it is impossible that diseased conditions of the pelvis and of the brain can have any dependence upon each other. Upon just such absurdities as these — for I can honestly apply to them no milder epithet — have many of the dogmas of psychologists been founded. As well might it be asserted, that because some persons with musket wounds have recovered, therefore a bullet never kills; or, because in some others, as in the late eminent geologist, Hugh Miller, for instance, extreme cerebral disorganization has, for a while, coexisted with apparent mental integrity, that, therefore, such disorganization is the normal condition of the brain, or can never be, at any rate, the cause of mental disturbance. And yet it is by just such baseless objections, that gentlemen, professing to seek only the advance of medicine and the cure of patients, have endeavored to prevent a more rational treatment of insane women than that now generally obtaining.

There are many questions directly presenting themselves in this connection, interesting equally in their practical and their scientific relations, upon which I have much to say, but whose discussion I must defer to another occasion. Such, among others, are the following: —

1. The effect of celibacy, of marriage, of widowhood, as causing insanity in women.

2. The transmissibility of insanity as an inheritance by the mother, as compared with it by the father.

3. The occurrence of uterine disease in the mother, as rendering the transmission of any family taint of insanity more probable to her offspring.

4. The frequency of organic cerebral disease in insane women as compared with it in insane men.*

5. The epidemics of Tarentism, convulsions, suicide, exhortation, &c., which, occurring among females, have at times so vexed the religious and profane worlds.

6. The special propensities of invalid women to breach of the law or of propriety, as in the so-called pyromania, klepto-, dipso-, erotomania; whether this last be for a real or imaginary object, and their responsibility therefor.

7. The possibilities of a longer incubation of insanity, from special causes, in invalid women than would probably be thought credible.

8. The periodicity of insanity in women, and the

---

* " Female insanity is in a large proportion of cases merely a reflex disturbance of the brain. Insanity in men much more extensively involves cerebral lesion, and their mortality is proportionately increased." Workman: Toronto Report, 1860; American Journal of the Medical Sciences, April, 1863, p. 437.

various lengths of the attack and the interval; in some instances bounded by a single catamenial period, in others by the space of gestation, of lying-in, of lactation, or the whole cycle of uterine life, from puberty to the final climacteric.

9. The time of development or explosion of an hereditary predisposition to insanity; its frequent coincidence with a special epoch in woman's life.

10. Epilepsy in women, with or without the addition of decided insanity, or its previous existence as a family taint, and the legal responsibilities of female epileptics.

I had prepared from my own note-books the histories of quite a number of cases, illustrating several of the special points now indicated, which I had intended here to present, in connection with the very interesting series published not long since by Dr. Azam, physician to the asylum for insane women at Bordeaux; but my paper is already so long that I must omit them. I cannot, however, refrain from quoting the last of Dr. Azam's conclusions, so completely does it coincide with my own conviction and my own experience.

"Every other treatment than physical will prove useless so long as the organic lesion persists, and this will have so much the greater chance of being effectual as it is resorted to at a time approaching the commencement of the disease." *

* De la folie sympathique provoquée et entretenue par les lésions de l'utérus et de ses annexes.

VIII. — Indications of Treatment.

My remarks, present and past, upon the causation of insanity in women have been elicited, as will long since have been perceived, by the need, as it seems to me, of urging upon the profession a more rational treatment, in public and private practice, of female lunatics. My views upon the subject are not the result of any hasty and ill-based impression, but they are matured, and from somewhat extensive observation. Without the slightest presumption, I think I may here say that I know whereof I do affirm. I cannot at this time go into the detail that I would gladly do, and that I have intended doing at no long subsequent period; but I shall at least show, as I think indeed I have already done, that the field now endeavored to be opened to the practical purposes of the profession is one that, though hitherto neglected, is yet one of the most fruitful in medicine.

As has hitherto been done in this communication, I shall endeavor to present the little I have time to say concerning treatment, through the language of superintendents themselves.

An author whom as yet I have hardly referred to, Dr. Conolly, of the asylum at Hanwell, while taking the general ground of non-restraint, seems to have been struck by the eminently sad condition, under the best of care, of lunatic women as compared with lunatic men. I cannot better introduce the little I can say in this especial connection, than by the following extract. Dr. Conolly says, —

"The precise condition of the brain in different patients is, it has been acknowledged, as little known as the mode and nature of its actions in health. The manner in which its functions are interrupted or disordered in insanity, lies in a region beyond the reach of man's senses, and seems scarcely a legitimate object for strictly philosophical imagination, unaided by any means of appreciating it, and leading merely to 'wandering thoughts and notions vain.' But the connection of these actions with material organs, and their evident sympathy with the body in health and in disease, impart certain resources to the physician, who, if he can only act directly on the mind within narrow limits, finds that he can extensively and powerfully influence it by sedulous attention to the state of the temple in which, in this condition of existence, it is enshrined." *

Let us see what until very lately has been this "sedulous attention to the state of the temple of the mind," so justly deemed necessary by Dr. Conolly. I shall first quote from an official English report of but a few years ago, with the simple comment that what then existed in Great Britain, still exists, to our disgrace, in many places in this country.

"In one of the cells for the women, the dimensions of which were eight feet by four, and in which there was no table, and only two wooden seats, we found three females confined. There was no glazing to the window, and the floor of the place was perfectly wet with urine. The two dark cells which joined the cell used for a day-room, are the sleeping places for these three unfortunate beings. Two of

---
* Treatment of the Insane, p. 164.

them sleep in two cribs in one cell. The floor in the cell with two cribs was actually reeking wet with urine, and covered with straw and filth. There is no window, and no place for light or air except a grate over the doors." *

Ten years later than the date of the report from which the above is quoted, it was my fortune to be residing in Scotland, when its lunatic asylums, public and private, were subjected to the official scrutiny that had been instigated by Miss Dix. The descriptions already given and to follow are in no respect an exaggeration of what, in many quarters, was found to exist. Among the foremost in promoting that investigation was my instructor, the late Professor Simpson; and it was the facts that then came to my knowledge, that first called my attention to the necessity of more thoroughly studying the causation and treatment of insanity in women. I will present a true picture from an unbiassed observer.

"The first common room you examine, measuring twelve feet long by seven wide, with a window which does not open, is [perhaps] for females. Ten of them, with no other covering than a rag round the waist, are chained to the wall, loathsome and hideous, but, when addressed, evidently retaining some of the intelligence, and much of the feeling, which, in other days, ennobled their nature. In shame or sorrow one of them perhaps utters a cry; a blow, which brings the blood from the temple, the tear from the eye, — an additional chain, a gag, and an indecent or contemptuous expression, produce silence. And if you ask where these creatures sleep, you are led to a kennel eight feet square,

* Report of the English Commissioners in Lunacy for 1844.

with an unglazed air-hole eight inches in diameter; in this, you are told, five women sleep. The floor is covered, the walls bedaubed, with filth and excrement: no bedding but wet, decayed straw is allowed; and the stench is so insupportable, that you turn away, and hasten from the scene."*

Dr. Conolly says, —

"Indeed, it would almost seem as if, at the period from the middle to near the end of the last century,† the superintendents of the insane had become frantic in cruelty, from the impunity with which their despotism was attended. Some of the German physicians meditated even romantic modes of alarm and torture; they wished for machinery, by which a patient, just arriving at an asylum, and after being drawn with frightful clangor over a metal bridge across a moat, could be suddenly raised to the top of a tower, and as suddenly lowered into a dark and subterranean cavern; and they avowed that if the patient could be made to alight among snakes and serpents it would be better still. People not naturally cruel became habituated to severity, until all feelings of humanity were forgotten. I used to be astonished, even seventeen years ago, to see humane physicians going daily round the wards of asylums, mere spectators of every form of distressing coercion, without a word of sympathy, or any order for its mitigation. But men's hearts had on this subject become gradually hardened. In medical works of authority, the first principle in the treatment of lunatics was laid down to be fear, and the best means of producing fear was said to be punishment, and the best mode of punishment was defined to be stripes. The great authority of Dr. Cullen, certainly one of the most enlightened physicians of his time, was given to this practice, although his theory of madness was, that it depended upon an increased excitement of the brain.

---

* Browne: What Asylums were, are, and ought to be. Edinburgh.
† We have seen that examples like those referred to have not entirely been unknown in the present century.

"Thus, by degrees, restraints became more and more severe, and torture more and more ingenious. Among many cruel devices, an unsuspecting patient was sometimes induced to walk across a treacherous floor; it gave way, and the patient fell into a bath of surprise, and was there half drowned and half frightened to death.*

"In some continental asylums the patients were chained in a well, and the water was allowed gradually to ascend, in order to terrify the patient with the prospect of inevitable death. Other methods adopted, even within the last sixty years, for controlling the phenomena of insanity, can only be regarded as tacit acknowledgments of the general inefficiency of medicine, and of the coarse determination of vain or ignorant men to effect by force what they could not accomplish by science. We read with almost as much amusement as wonder the respectful acknowledgment of Dr. Hallaran, that Dr. Cox made known to the profession the 'safe and effectual remedy' of the circulating swing, the invention of which Dr. Cox 'generously gives the credit of' to Dr. Darwin; this invention being one by means of which the maniacal or melancholic patient, fast bound on a sort of couch, or in a chair, was rotated at various rates up to one hundred gyrations in a minute. This machine was used with two indications; the horizontal position being adopted when the object was to procure sleep; and the erect posture, the other failing, in cases of excitement, to procure intestinal action. It is acknowledged that patients once subjected to the swing were ever afterwards terrified at the mention of it; that it lowered the pulse and the temperature to such a degree as to alarm the physician; that it occasioned a 'disagreeable suffusion of the countenance,' frequently leaving an ecchymosis of the eyes; that it acted as an emetic, and as a hypercathartic; but still it was lauded as reducing the unmanageable, and, stranger still, as causing the melan-

---

* It was with reference to this bath of surprise, which was said to have effected actual cures, that Esquirol remarked, justly enough, "I should as soon think of recommending patients to be precipitated from the third story of a house, because some lunatics have been known to be cured by a fall on the head."

choly to take 'a natural interest in the affairs of life.' It is curious to be told, also, that the inconvenient effects mentioned were induced more certainly when the patient was in the erect position. Worse consequences occasionally resulted, I believe, from this barbarous invention; which probably rendered Dr. Hallaran's recommendation, that no 'well-regulated institution, intended for the reception and relief of insane persons,' should be unprovided with a machine of that description, ineffectual. Allusion is made to the practice in Esquirol's work,* in which he describes 'la machine de Darwin' as resembling the *jeu de bague*, or treadmill, and he speaks of it as having passed from the arts into medicine. It found some temporary favor on the continent; but the violent evacuations produced by its employment, followed by fainting and excessive debility, led to its disuse. Dr. Cox had advised its being used in some 'hopeless' cases, in the dark, with the addition of unusual noises, smells, etc., that every sense might be assailed; but I do not think that this advice was ever acted upon." †

In the women's galleries in Bethlem, the same author tells us, they found in one of the side rooms "about ten patients, each chained by one arm or leg to the wall; the chain allowing them merely to stand up by the bench or form fixed to the wall, or to sit down on it." For a dress, each had only a sort of a blanket-gown, made like a dressing-gown, but with nothing to fasten it round the body. The feet were without shoes or stockings. Some of these patients were lost in imbecility, dirty, and offensive; associated with them were others capable of coherent conversation, and sensible, and accomplished. Many women were locked up in their cells, chained, with-

* Conolly, pp. 12-15. † Loc. cit., vol. i. p. 156.

out clothing, and with only one blanket for a covering.*

"At that time, when a young and accomplished woman, for example, affected with acute mania, violent, noisy, mischievous, regardless of cleanliness, arrived at a large asylum, she was forcibly undressed, fastened down on loose straw, had strong medicine forced down her throat, and was then left and neglected for many hours. The straw tortured her from head to foot, but she could not move her hands. Her position galled and fretted her; but her feet were fastened, and she could not change it. Sickness and purging were produced by the medicine; and she was permitted to lie for twelve hours in a state of indescribable distress, then taken up, laid on the stone pavement, mopped or broomed, and, last of all, when quite subdued and half dead, had, perhaps, a bath and some few decent attentions." †

And again : —

"The history of each patient, and the afflictions which had caused their minds to give way, would now receive attention in all good asylums. But the day had not arrived for such kind sympathies, and on arriving at the large and crowded house the patient was undressed, with small show of gentleness, by several young women, and placed at once in a crib, on straw, and fastened to it by the feet, her hands being confined by iron hand-locks, and a tight waistcoat put around the trunk of the body and round her arms, the offices of the nurses concluding for the time with the administration of a dose of purgative salts. When the patient, not yet forgetful of the decencies of life, asked what she was to do if she wanted to get out of bed, the nurses, hardened by their vocation, merely answered her in the most vulgar terms. Having, in this miserable restraint, become dirty, which was inevitable, the patient was taken out of bed, carried to the pump, and pumped upon with cold water, and then, un-

* Loc. cit., p. 26. † Ibid., p. 48.

dried, taken back to her crib, and fastened down again, but on fresh straw ; an attention not then in all cases considered necessary. All her remonstrances to the women about her were laughed at. Long afterwards she still remembered her own expressions and theirs, her appeals to them as women, her prayers for pity, and their too ready reply, which shut out hope — 'You don't know what a mad-house is yet, but we will teach you.' In the same room there were, she remembered, several maniacs, all in chains or restraints of some kind, singing, swearing, beating the walls. This scene, and her aggravated wretchedness, made her worse; and as she could not get up and move about, she could only sing or shout aloud like the rest. For six weeks she was kept in that place of torment, and in those restraints; and, like most of the patients of those old asylums, the story of her restraints was written in broad indelible scars on her wrists, but in still worse characters on her memory." *

That such abuses, thus related by a superintendent himself, were more common with women than with men, there can be no question. It is still so, to the degree, more or less marked as this may be, to which they still exist. And there are reasons why it might be expected that such should be the case, as is implied by the author from whom we have been quoting. Dr. Conolly says, —

"On the female side of the house, where the greatest daily amount of excitement and refractoriness was to be met and managed, the cases of recent insanity in young women, and especially the cases of puerperal insanity, and those arising from lactation, were, perhaps, the first to attract particular notice in reference to the new system. Anywhere but where restraints are indiscriminately employed, such cases would seem the likeliest to be regarded with

---

* Loc. cit., p. 124.

interest and compassion, and to be treated with gentleness. But as they are usually attended with a great degree of excitement, and with a lively propensity to every kind of mischief, and consequently occasion much trouble, these cases had become more especially and constantly subjected to severe coercion.*

"The subjects of this coercion were, some of them, women of middle age, who had been handsome, and who possessed considerable acuteness of intellect, ingenuity, and activity, but whose lives had been a sort of troubled romance; profligate, intemperate, violent, regardless of domestic ties, their children abandoned to all the evils of homeless poverty, themselves by degrees given up to utter recklessness, they had been the cause of ruin and shame to their families, and the history of their wild life had closed with madness. Others, and not a few, were the victims of the vices of those of a station superior to them, and left at length to struggle with difficulties, and mortifications, and remorse, beneath which reason gave way. In these patients all violent methods produced greater obstinacy, greater determination to give trouble, to do mischief, and to commit all kinds of outrages.†

"Delicate young women, affected with mania, were tied to the bed, or half-smothered by servant-women and men, or fastened down by sheets twisted into the shape of cables, and tightly bound round the body and round the bed. In this miserable condition cleanliness is neglected, and the patient suffers from heat and thirst, and becomes exhausted by vain struggles. The patient becomes rapidly emaciated and perfectly frantic. Nothing can allay the irritation created by the useless crowd, by the disorder of the room, and the closeness of the atmosphere, and all the horrors which in the course of a few dreadful days have been needlessly accumulated about the chamber of a patient laboring under an excited brain, and whose malady all these things do but increase. But in these unhappy cases the friends still often

---

* Loc. cit., p. 107. † Ibid., p. 127.

oppose measures of a different kind, preferring the absolute secrecy thrown over the malady before all sensible considerations. Their prejudices and weakness find support in the arguments or insinuations of the attendants, who are glad to be relieved from trouble, and who commonly neglect to provide against any danger, except by debarring the patient from muscular movement as much as possible, and as long as possible. If, happily, such cases are transferred to the care of attendants who have been taught not to rely upon, or even to have recourse to, restraints, the alteration effected in a day or two is such as to make it difficult to believe that the patient is the same person seen before. If the patient is removed from home to a tranquil asylum, the change is greater still. At home the patient is, perhaps, the cause of indescribable confusion : all domestic regularity is interrupted, the servants speak in whispers, the neighbors avoid the house. Days and nights are passed in anxiety or terror. But the patient who has unconsciously caused all this disturbance becomes, when taken to an asylum conducted on good principles, quite an altered person; disturbing nobody, and behaving peaceably, and even seeming happy among new associates, and in scenes unconnected with the real or imaginary griefs of the home so lately quitted. Such sudden improvement certainly almost exceeds belief; but the instances of it are not even rare. Every physician conversant with practice in cases of insanity, must have witnessed these almost marvellous metamorphoses many times." *

Let it not be supposed that the fearful pictures I have now shown of the attention paid the most sacred of human temples by medical men are either overdrawn or from a wholly by-gone age. They merely represent what I have myself witnessed upon more than one occasion here in Massachusetts within

* Loc. cit., p. 329.

the past few years. Such cases, resulting from the neglect or omission of the profession to prevent their occurrence, become in reality acts of commission upon its part. I make no reflection upon the management of asylums, for it is well known that gross abuses of the kind described are no longer permitted to occur therein; but there are hundreds of insane women in each of our States, some of whom have already been in hospitals, others of whom have never received even the partial and necessarily imperfect examination it is there customary to make, who are now under treatment outside these hospitals, or rather under no medical treatment whatever, but subject only to the brutalities of the town's officials who have them in charge. For further evidence upon this subject, I need merely refer to the report of the Commission of which I was then a member.* If such outrages still exist in Massachusetts, there is reason to believe they are not wholly unknown in other States of the Union,† and it is the duty of the profession to look to it that they are at once made to cease.

I would not, however, while allowing the prevention at hospitals of the open abuse of female patients, be understood to admit that all is there accomplished

---

* Report of the Commissioners (Quincy, Hitchcock, and H. R. Storer) on Insanity to the Legislature of Massachusetts. Pub. Doc. 1864, Senate, No. 72.
† The facts in the case are but too patent. They were acknowledged to exist in two other States at the moment the above was written (American Journal of Insanity, Jan., 1865). They undoubtedly exist in every State of the Union.

that might and ought to be done. Far from this. Neglect, systematic and customary though it may be, of any means or measure that may tend to the cure of a patient, or a class of patients, is in reality almost as grievous a wrong as a harm intentionally inflicted. Between omission and commission there is at times but very little difference as regards the injury that is done.

Let me here quote, as pertinent to this question, from a late report of the State Hospital for the Insane of California — a report characterized by Dr. Earle, of the Northampton Asylum, as " essentially different in character from any other from the California hospital which has come under our observation, its particular object appearing to be an exposition of the defects of the hospital as a curative establishment." *

" Its beautiful edifice," says Dr. Tilden, the superintendent, " its well-cultivated yards and gardens, its wholesome food, its comfortable clothing, its scrupulously clean halls, rooms, beds, and bedding, its excellent police regulations, combine in making a prison of the first class; and, if such was the original purpose, I see not how it could have been more admirably accomplished. If, however, in creating a charity so munificent, so noble, it was intended to establish an asylum, with hospital appliances, for the *cure*, as well as the care and safe-keeping of the insane, I am

* American Journal of the Medical Sciences, April, 1865, p. 445

free to say it is, in my opinion, a most signal failure.' And again, he says, "If there is any marked difference between it and a well-conducted State prison, it is in favor of the latter, from the fact that means of employment are provided for its inmates, while the inmates of the asylum spend their days in idleness." And again, "It will hardly be contended, I think, that our newspapers and a little gymnasium, with a solitary swing in the female department, can give the asylum of California a claim to the character of a curative institution."

"The general use of mechanical restraint," says Dr. Tuke, "arose from the idea impressed upon the keepers of asylums, no less by the highest authorities than by a venerable antiquity, that it was the necessary and best mode of treatment. It was connected," he continues, "with a theoretical ignorance of the nature and pathology of insanity."* The same should be said of the neglect to extend to an insane woman the same method of examination and of treatment which would be considered imperative for the same woman laboring under any other possibly reflex form of disease.

I have quoted upon this point the pithy corollary of Dr. Azam, that for organic causative disease, physical means only are effectual; and I have given the corroborative testimony of Dr. Tuke, regarding the

---

* Manual of Psychological Medicine, p. 76.

chronic and supposed incurable cases of insanity in women now at the Morningside Asylum. Let me submit a word or two in addition from still other superintendents. We are told that, —

"With regard to the detection of internal disease, great care is required, as many of those symptoms on which the practitioner generally relies as aids to diagnosis are wholly suppressed. Insane persons frequently evince either great insensibility to, or power of enduring pain, and hence the light afforded by painful and morbid sensations is absent in the internal and constitutional diseases affecting persons of unsound mind. From this cause, examinations after death occasionally reveal organic lesions and changes which had not previously been supposed to exist, and it requires careful attention to the physical signs present, and a close observation of disordered functions and constitutional peculiarities, in order to discover the disease which is, perhaps, secretly undermining the vital powers.*

"In the purely medical aspects of the subject," it has been remarked by the same author, "there appears in some quarters an indolent and ultra-expectant mode of regarding mental diseases, which, if pursued to its legitimate consequences, must end in the utter repudiation of medical science and skill in their treatment. For in the reports of some large asylums, I observe that medical treatment is intimated to be of little avail, one or two drugs being mentioned as the only medicinal agencies employed. If this be the correct principle, if medical science can afford no greater aid in the cure of insanity, it is surely incumbent on the medical officers who entertain these views at once to resign their appointments as such, and henceforth leave the care of the insane to persons of ordinary education. For my own part I entertain a very different opinion. I believe that even in this apparently unpromising department of medicine great results may be achieved; and that by a more

---

* Robinson: **Prevention and Treatment of Mental Disorders**, p. 183.

perfect acquaintance with the laws regulating the phenomena of the healthy mind, by a more extended knowledge of the properties of the innumerable substances, natural and artificial, which are capable of acting upon the nervous structures, and through them upon the mental phenomena, and by a more careful investigation of the circumstances influencing the production of morbid changes in the nervous system, a merely disordered and structurally uninjured brain may be rendered as amenable to curative agencies as a disordered liver or kidney." *

Bucknill says, —

" The medicinal treatment, therefore, must be founded, not upon the general resemblance of symptoms in different cases,† but upon their points of dissemblance, and upon the discrimination of ultimate diagnosis; not the primary diagnosis which recognizes a case of insanity, but upon the ultimate diagnosis which, as nearly as possible, refers the symptoms of each individual case to the exact pathological condition from which they arise." ‡

Esquirol exclaims, —

" What misfortunes and obstacles must those practitioners have encountered who have been only able to see one individual disease in all the insanities which they have had to treat! They were not ignorant that, delirium being symptomatic of almost all diseases when approaching a fatal termination, insanity might be also entirely symptomatic; they were not ignorant that there are instances of insanity evidently sympathetic; they knew that a thousand exciting and predisposing causes give rise to insanity; but paying no attention except to the most obvious symptoms, they have permitted themselves to be imposed upon by the impetuosity, the violence, the mobility of these; they have neglected the study of the causes of insanity, and that of the relation of the causes with the symptoms. Under the domination

---

* Robinson: Prevention and Treatment of Mental Disorders, p. 225.
† It will be noticed what a blow is this remark to the usual system of classification of the insane. ‡ Loc. cit., p 453.

of theories, some have only been able to see the existence of inflammation, have accused the blood, and abused the lancet; others, believing in irritating bile, have checked the secreting organs, and injured their functions. They have been prodigal of emetics and drastics. Some, having only taken into account the nervous influence, have given antispasmodics in excess. All have forgotten that the practitioner ought to have present to his mind grand general views — the systematic ideas which dominate, which constitute medical science, the art which ought especially to devote itself to a thorough knowledge of the circumstances, and of the symptoms, which are capable of disclosing the causes, the seat, and the nature of the malady which it has to combat. Often one must vary, combine, modify the means of treatment; for there is no specific treatment of insanity. As this malady is not identical in all persons, so it has in every individual its different causes and characters; so new combinations are required, and a new problem is to be solved for each insane person under treatment." *

What grand general views, let me ask, what systematic ideas, what search for different causes and characters, and for new combinations, the resort to what means of solving the problem, do we find in the usual and most ancient method of treating insane women? That I am neither doing injustice by this question, nor venturing an opinion without a sufficient reason, I may be permitted to refer the profession to extended papers by leading authorities upon the subject, who may be supposed to have given a fair statement of the present methods of medically treating the insane. As instances in point, I will name Dr. Forbes Winslow's articles on the Treatment of In-

* Maladies Mentales.

sanity, Ancient and Modern,* and on the Medical Treatment of Insanity; † those by Schrœder van der Kolk, ‡ even the excellent one to which I have already referred in another part of this report, and that by Dr. Ranney, Physician to the City Lunatic Asylum of New York,§ which enjoyed the honor of being reproduced, with the full discussion to which it gave rise at the meeting of American Superintendents, to whom it was first communicated, in one of the English psychological journals. ‖ In none of them do we find recognition of the claims of a decided and special treatment for insane women, although, in the case of Winslow, it will be recollected that he had acknowledged the special causation of much of their mental disturbance, as suggested by Laycock.

I would not deny the occurrence in psychological literature of sentences like the following, for I have already quoted many of them; but they have as yet fallen without fruit, and dead. "Sex," says Dr. Robertson, "is doubtless an indication of treatment in the many cases connected with uterine disease." ¶

Dr. Conolly, as usual, here speaks sensibly and intelligibly.

* Journal of Psychological Medicine, Jan., 1850.
† Ibid, April, 1854.
‡ British and Foreign Medico-Chirurgical Review; American Journal of Insanity, July, 1860.
§ Ibid; July, 1857.
‖ Asylum Journal of Mental Science, April, 1858, p. 450.
¶ Ibid., Jan., 1859, p. 277.

"The physician's office is assuming in these times a higher character in proportion as he ceases to be a mere prescriber of medicines, and acts as the guardian or conservator of public and of private health; studious of all agencies that influence the body and the mind, and which, affecting individual comfort and longevity, act widely on societies of human beings. Changes are gradually taking place even in special walks of medical practice, in conformity to the enlightened principles by which the exertions of the officers of general health are directed; and these principles find an application, and are strikingly illustrated, in the modern asylums and modern treatment of the insane. Obscurity may yet hang over the origin of mental derangement; the explanation of sudden recoveries may continue difficult; the alterations incidental to portions of nervous matter may baffle investigation, and the possible varieties in the condition of the blood, often apparently associated with mental disturbance, may be yet unknown, or incapable of satisfactory elucidation; but general means have been revealed to men of science, conducing to important modifications and ameliorations of mental malady." *

It is possible that I may be able to afford some light as to the frequency with which these means are at present resorted to in the case of insane women. I have spoken of the neglect of special measures, as in reality the prevalent treatment of insane women. Of such a method as is the present, Dr. Bucknill speaks as follows: —

"Although specific drugs are out of vogue, narrow and stereotyped modes of treatment are scarcely less dangerous; and in no class of disease does the treatment need to be more infinitely varied than in insanity. In other wide classes, some broad rules may be laid down for the treat-

* Treatment of the Insane, p. 79.

ment; and although physicians may differ respecting these rules, they will be found to adhere to one or other set of opinions respecting them. Thus, one feeds in fevers, another depletes; but in insanity, cases which present symptoms, at first sight, of close resemblance, demand most opposite modes of treatment; and cases which at first present symptoms most unlike, sometimes require to be treated in the same manner. An educated and exact observation is required to distinguish between the acute delirium which arises from cerebral hyperæmia and that which arises from cerebral excitement in sympathy with intense irritation of some part of the periphery of the nervous system; or from the cerebral excitement which is but an expression of the defective nutrition of the organ from poverty of the blood; or cerebral excitement propagated to all parts of the organ from some focus of irritation, some *foyer* of disease in itself, as a small portion of inflamed substance or membrane, or the structural mischiefs surrounding an apoplectic clot. In all these instances the symptoms may bear a strong resemblance to each other, and yet how different is the mode of treatment demanded in each of them." *

It has been asserted, that in claiming for insane women the same general principles of treatment by which we would conduct disease to a successful issue where the mind is unimpaired, I am myself endeavoring to substitute for the present general neglect a narrow and stereotyped method of practice. Every one familiar with the modern treatment of the diseases of women, will detect and deny this wretched libel. It is just the man who does not treat symptoms, but searches faithfully and persistently for their ultimate cause, who is the true general practitioner —

* Loc. cit., p. 452.

he, alone, who can avoid the charge of blind groping and routine.

In one of my previous communications upon insanity as of reflex causation in women, the statement was made, with all respect for the ability and zeal of those more especially engaged in the management of the insane, that little has as yet been undertaken or accomplished at our public hospitals for the cure of insane women.

" Does he mean to say," asks an anonymous critic, whom I have noticed only because he claims to have been both Assistant Physician and Superintendent of a New England Asylum, and to represent the opinion of a large circle of his fraternity—"does he mean to say that superintendents have not discharged, as cured, as many women as men? Where are the statistics?"*

To the statistics thus called for, although I have already in this communication expressed an emphatic belief as to their real value, I am yet not unwilling to refer.

I should have produced them ere this, had I not preferred that they should be called for by any gentleman who might venture to deny the justice of my conclusions. Those who appeal to statistics, cannot refuse to be governed by their evidence.

I proceed to draw additional proof of the correct

---

* Boston Medical and Surgical Journal, 5th January, 1865, p 453 ness of my views concerning the management of insane women: —

A. From the statistical evidence of asylums, and

B. From the direct evidence of those having asylums in charge.*

A. In the first place, I would say that any remarks I may have made respecting the medical management of insane women at asylums, apply not merely to our own American hospitals, but to those of other countries also — so that no argument in disproof can be drawn from the comparisons I shall proceed to furnish, inasmuch as these, being based upon nearly identical data, can only afford identical results.

Secondly, I have no doubt, and I am willing to allow, that as many, or nearly as many women as men are yearly discharged from asylums. Any basis that may be named, the number of admissions, for instance, may be taken for the calculation. Selecting

* A portion of the evidence that will now be presented was read before the Suffolk District Medical Society of Boston on January 28, 1865. It was communicated to the Medical and Surgical Journal of that city as Article IV. of the series I had already initiated, upon the causation and treatment of insanity in women; the subject being one whose discussion many of the most distinguished physicians in this country are pleased to consider of the very highest importance. On the 15th of February I received the following note: "The editors of the Journal came to the conclusion, after the publication of the last article relating to this discussion, that enough space had already been given to it, and that they would decline any further communication on the subject." With this decision I have not found fault, the gentlemen referred to best understanding their own affairs. So many inquiries, however, concerning my enforced silence have been made of me by their subscribers who had seen my former papers, and by the gentlemen who were present at the reading of that herein embodied, that I should certainly have published through some other medium the facts here presented, had they not been so relevant to the main subject of the present report.

at random from a pile of hospital reports, I will give the results of the statistics of the Worcester State Hospital for the space of thirty years, from 1833–62. In a total of over 6000 patients, there were admitted 3273 males and 3390 females, and were discharged 2962 males, or 88 per cent. of the admissions, and 3078 females, or 89 per cent. of the admissions, a difference of 1 per cent. in favor of the women.

If we add the years 1863 and '64, the percentage is but slightly changed. In a total of over 7000 patients, we now have as admitted 3503 males and 3601 females, and as discharged 2910 males, or 81 per cent. of the admissions, a loss of 7 per cent., and 3005 females, or 81 per cent. of the admissions, a loss of 8 per cent.; the proportions of discharges in the two sexes being rendered exactly identical by the comparative loss of 1 per cent. by the women.

Thirdly, I have also no doubt, and am willing to admit, that as many, or nearly as many women as men are discharged from our hospitals as recovered. This, it will be noticed, is, however, a very different thing from being discharged as cured; and this again is by no means identical with being discharged cured.

If my views as to the psycho-pathology of women are correct, not only as many women as men ought to be discharged cured, but very many more. This, however, does not occur in practice.

To return to the question of relative recoveries. At

the Worcester State Hospital, during the thirty years first mentioned, and upon the basis of admissions then existing, namely, 3273 males and 3390 females, there were discharged as recovered, 1493 males, or 44 per cent. of the admissions, and 1618 females, or 45 per cent. of the admissions; a difference of 1 per cent. in favor of the females.

Adding again the years 1863 and '64, we have an admission of 3503 males and 3601 females, and a discharge as recovered, of 1612 males, or 45 per cent. of the admissions, a gain of 1 per cent., and 1751 females, or 49 per cent. of the admissions, a gain of 4 per cent.; showing a difference of 4 per cent. in the females, and a comparative gain of 3 per cent.

At the Southern Ohio Lunatic Asylum, for the nine years from 1855–64, there were admitted 497 males and 499 females; of whom were discharged as recovered, 261 males, or 57 per cent. of the admissions, and 251 females, or 50 per cent. of the admissions; a proportion of 7 per cent. in favor of the males.

At the Taunton State Hospital, for the nine years from 1853–62, there were admitted 1044 males and 1004 females, and were discharged as recovered 404 males, or 38 per cent. of the admissions, and 335 females, or 30 per cent. of the admissions; a proportion of 8 per cent. in favor of the males.

If we tabulate the results of these three hospitals, we have for the years first considered, a total of nearly

10,000 patients admitted, of whom 4814 were males, and 4933 were females. Of the former there were discharged as recovered 2158, or 42 per cent., and of the latter 2204, or 44 per cent.; a difference of 2 per cent. in favor of the female.

Adding to this the years 1863 and '64 at the Worcester Asylum, our total number of patients admitted becomes 12,000; 6844 being males, and 5104 females. There were discharged as recovered 2277 males, or 31 per cent., a loss of 11 per cent., and 2337 females, or 44 per cent., the proportion here remaining the same. The difference of 13 per cent. which had been relatively gained by the women, and which at first sight might have seemed an absolute gain, being found upon comparison to be exactly neutralized by the loss in recoveries of the men.

The statistics that have now been given were, as I have said, taken at random from many reports before me, and may undoubtedly be considered as representing the truth, *such as it is*. They show, it will be noticed, an apparent variation of the ratio of recoveries in insane women at the different hospitals — ranging from 50 per cent. at Dayton to 30 per cent. at Taunton — a variation to be explained in part, by the different probable character and nationality of the patients at the two hospitals; if at all attributable to difference in treatment, it may partly be owing to the fact, as is well known, that Dr. Gundry has paid much attention to insanity as caused by or coincident with the puerperal state. These variations, however, but tend to make the mean that I have presented the more reliable in reference to the actual percentage of recoveries of insane women at asylums.

I could have furnished a computation upon a very much larger scale had it been necessary; that given is, however, sufficient for every practical purpose, more especially as I have granted all that could by any one be claimed; namely, that at our hospitals as many insane women as men are discharged as recovered.

It will not be uninteresting, however, to compare these results with what obtains abroad; a comparison that so far as I am aware has never yet been made.

At the York Retreat, in England, as appears from a table furnished by Tuke, and covering a period of 51 years, from 1796 to 1857, the average proportion of recoveries as compared with the admissions was 49.54 per cent. of males and 49.50 per cent. of females, the numbers being almost exactly identical.[*]

It was Dr. Thurnam's opinion, as we have already seen, that the proportion of recoveries of women exceeded those of men by about 20 per cent.; indeed, he is said to have estimated this excess as high as 50 per cent. A most surprising difference as compared with the results I am now presenting.

[*] Psychological Medicine, p. 201.

At Bethlem, during ten years, 53.8 per cent. of the men recovered, and 54.4 per cent. of the women; an excess of .6 per cent. in favor of the latter.*

At St. Yon, near Rouen, in France, the difference in favor of the women has been rated at 3 per cent. †

In most of the French asylums it has been thought that the males, discharged as recovered, exceeded the females by about 6 per cent. It is possible, however, that in some instances these computations may have been made by comparison with the total number of discharges, as was the case in the English statistical tables presented by Farr. The excess referred to has been noticed by nearly all the directors of asylums in France, and has been explained in various ways. By some it is regarded as due to "a humane sentiment, which induces the physicians of these establishments to shorten as much as possible the period of confinement for the men, whose labor is oftentimes indispensable to the maintenance of their families; and, on the other hand, to detain the females, giving them the protection of the asylum as long as possible, in view of their greater helplessness, and of the dangers to which many would be exposed on their return to society;" a detention which, besides, by preventing to a certain extent their marriage, would tend to check the

---

* Hood: Statistics of Bethlem Hospital, p. 73; as corrected by Tuke, loc. cit., p. 262.

† Parchappe: Notice Statistique sur les Aliénés de la Seine Inferieure, p. 44

transmission of a predisposition to the disease by inheritance.

"But," says Legoyt, "ought we not rather to attribute this difference to the greater or less severity of the disease itself, depending upon the difference in causes which induce insanity in the two sexes?"*

I allow the validity of the explanation by which the apparent disparity is done away, calling attention only to the admission that insanity in the two sexes may be owing to a constantly frequent difference in cause.

Thus far, it has been shown that the discharges of women from hospitals, as recovered, is about equal to that of men. Let it not be supposed, however, that this is necessarily a proof that, 1st, these recoveries are always cures; 2d, that they comprise all the women who might be cured; or, 3d, that they are evidence that all justifiable resources of medical treatment have been put in requisition.

I propose, on the contrary, by pursuing the investigation a little further, to show the opposite.

1. Are these recoveries always cures? It is a delicate question that I am now approaching; but I rely upon the good nature of those interested in the matter who are my personal friends, and upon the fairness of all others, that they take no offence where none is intended.

* American Journal of Insanity, April, 1861, p. 424.

In view of the coincidence already shown to exist, as regards the relative recoveries of the two sexes in asylums, at home and abroad, I may be permitted to seek evidence from foreign sources, inasmuch as minute data have not yet been afforded to any extent from within our own asylums. An identity of result may of course be supposed to have been occasioned by similarity of cause.

At some foreign establishments, nearly one third of all the patients treated are set down as cures, while in others only three or four per cent. of the recoveries are claimed as the result of treatment.* As this statement is given from Legoyt's statistics, by his translator, the well-known physician to the Long Island Asylum at Sanford Hall, without objection or other comment, the fact is probably not materially different from what may be supposed to obtain in this country also.† No exception seems to have been taken to the statement by any other of our writers on insanity during the nearly four years (1865) since these statistics were reproduced by Dr. Barstow.

The difference, to which I have referred, is supposed to be due partly to accidental circumstances, appearing and disappearing at different asylums at different periods of time, partly to the diversity of curative measures or of the hygienic conditions by

---

* Deductions from the Statistics of the Establishments for the Insane in France, for the twelve years from 1842 to 1853 inclusive.
† American Journal of Insanity, April, 1861, p. 423.

which patients are surrounded, and partly to the longer or shorter period of residence at the asylum which each physician may order as requisite for his patient.

"This may be done on the part of the physician as a result of enlightened experience and observation, or in view sometimes of the material interests of the institution of which he has the charge. We may suppose, for example, that where the number of beds is found inadequate to the wants of the service, and where maintenance of a very large number of patients is at the public expense, their discharge is more easily authorized at the first well-marked symptoms of returning health, than where such maintenance is a source of income to the establishment."*

It is allowed, then, by alienists of acknowledged authority, that these so-called recoveries are not *always* cures. Are they generally so? Before entering upon this question, evidence may be interesting as to what has been supposed the curability of the insane, positive and comparative, as to sex.

In the report of the Massachusetts Commissioners on Lunacy for 1854–55, which is a model of statistical research, it is stated that there were of insane men, native and foreign, in Massachusetts, 1259; and of insane women, 1373. Of the men, 181 were considered curable, and 1005 incurable; leaving 73 unaccounted for. Of the women, 225 were considered curable, and 999 incurable; leaving 149 unaccounted

---

* American Journal of Insanity, April, 1861, p. 423.

for.* Or, in other words, 14 per cent. of the men were considered curable, against the 44 per cent. discharged as recovered from the Worcester Hospital; and 16 per cent. of the women, against 45 per cent. These facts are the more interesting, as the writer of that report was also a Trustee of the State Hospital at Worcester, whose statistics have therefore undoubtedly passed under his own careful scrutiny.

It may be urged that this is hardly a fair basis for comparisons, as Dr. Jarvis's estimates were of the whole insane in Massachusetts, whether at hospitals or at home. Fortunately, he has provided us with other and more pertinent elements of computation. At the time referred to, 1854–55, there were in the Massachusetts hospitals for the insane, 522 men and 619 women. Of the men, 85, or 16 per cent., were considered curable; and of the women, 109, or 17 per cent.; the ratios being almost identically the same.† Is it proper, then, to compare these two classes of statistics — the proportion of discharges as recovered, with the whole number of admissions; and the considered curable, with the whole number at the hospitals? In view of their apparently constant character, I think it should be allowed. It may be urged that the number of incurable insane permanently resident at our hospitals invalidates any calcu-

---

* Report on Insanity and Idiocy in Massachusetts, 1855. House Doc. No. 144, p. 78.
† Ibid.

lation from which they are not eliminated; but, on the other hand, it may be judged, from the constant character of the statistics I have already given, that this number is also constant; and, besides, who has ever given us a standard by which to judge, or by which he has judged, of the incurability of insane women?

From the evidence given, it would appear that while some 44 per cent. of the women entering our hospitals are annually discharged as recovered, but 16 per cent. of the women at these hospitals were considered by the competent authority whom I have quoted, as at that time subjects of probable cure.

It is possible, however, that Dr. Jarvis intended the word *curability* as synonymous with capability of recovery. What is this capability of recovery of insane women?

In women, as in men, it has been seen that of all admitted to asylums, nearly one half are discharged well or much improved. A very marked difference, however, will be found to exist between the sexes, if we compare the age, not of the patients, but of their disease.

At the French asylums, it has been observed that for the first six months of asylum treatment, the recoveries of males exceed those of females, while for the next six months, on the contrary, the proportion is much greater for females than for males.* Dr. Tuke has given, from the statistics of the York Retreat, a table that throws much light upon this subject. Like one of those that I have already presented, it is computed from a period of sixty-one years.†

	Proportion of Recoveries.	
Duration of disorder when admitted.	Men.	Women.
First attack, and within three months,	72.97	73.23
" from three to twelve months,	43.07	44.20
Not first attack, and within twelve months,	59.44	67.01
First or not, and more than twelve months,	13.29	22.59

From the above, it appears that in the first of the classes named, the excess of recoveries in women was .26 per cent.; in the second class, 1.13 per cent.; in the third class, 7.57 per cent.; and in the fourth class, 9.30 per cent.

From sheets of the First Annual Report of the Massachusetts Board of State Charities, that were kindly afforded me, in advance of publication, by the Secretary, F. B. Sanborn, Esq., I was enabled to establish a computation to somewhat the same effect, namely, that while in acute and sudden, or explosive attacks of insanity, the percentages of recoveries in the sexes are at present nearly identical, in chronic cases there is quite a balance in favor of the women. Thus, at the Worcester Hospital, during the thirty-two years of its existence, there have been —

---

* Legoyt, loc. cit., p. 426.   † Loc. cit., p. 261.

IN WOMEN.

Standing of Disease.	Discharged recovered.		Percentage to Admissions.	
	Males.	Females.	Males.	Females.
1 year or less, . .	1242	1372	.55	.54
1 to 2 years, numbers not corresponding with each other, as reported.*				
2 to 5 years, . .	112	124	.22	.24
5 to 10 " . .	42	53	.15	.20
10 to 15 " . .	12	20	.8	.13
15 to 20 " . .	9	9	.13	.21
20 to 25 " . .	7	6	.14	.18

Beyond the limit last named, recoveries practically cease. It appears, then, that in the first of these periods the proportions of recovery between the two sexes was almost identical; in the second and third, there was an excess of 2 per cent. in favor of the women; in the fourth, of 5 per cent.; in the fifth, of 5 per cent.; in the sixth, of 8 per cent.; and in the last, of 4 per cent.

It is very much to be regretted that the tables, calculated in the Report of the Board of State Charities, which I have just quoted, drawn from the statistics of the Taunton Hospital, do not contain a statement of the relative numbers of the two sexes discharged as recovered, and of the relative numbers of admissions in the several periods stated, as I should thus have been able to have compared the statistics of the two hospitals more closely, and then, by combining them,

---

* First Annual Report of the Massachusetts Board of State Charities, p. 106. In the printed tables from which I have deduced these computations, there is given as discharged, recovered, not recovered, or dead, of the class referred to above, a total of 458 patients, male and female, out of only 227 admissions.

have procured a much larger, and therefore much more reliable, basis.*

Again, the relative mortality of the two sexes at asylums is very different, or, as it has been expressed by the director of an asylum, "the dangers and discomforts attending a residence in an insane asylum have a much less effect upon females than upon males." Thus, the smallest proportion of male deaths, reported at the French hospitals, during the twelve years whose statistics we have examined, was 15 per cent., while of females the minimum mortality was but 12 per cent.†

The average mortality during the whole of this period was in males, 54 per cent., and in females, 45 per cent.; the whole number of deaths being over 32,000, of which 17,390 were males, and 14,709 were

---

* With reference to this discrepancy, to which I have above adverted, Mr. Sanborn writes me as follows: "The number *discharged* recovered, after an insanity of from one to two years, would naturally be greater than the number *admitted* with insanity of the same duration; since of those admitted with insanity of less than one year's duration, a great many are not discharged until their malady has continued beyond a year.

"With regard to the want of uniformity in the tables referred to, you must remember that I have not attempted to go beyond the tables given by each superintendent. That would involve an amount of labor which you can, doubtless, appreciate, but which it has not been in the power of this department hitherto to perform. It is to be regretted that the superintendents do not agree upon a form of statistical record which will admit of perfect comparisons."

† American Journal of Insanity, April, 1861, p. 433. Dr. Barstow copies Legoyt's error of considering that these figures show an advantage for the women of 39 per cent. I have, however, detected the source of this fallacy in the punctuating of the decimals. Instead of .39, the calculation should have showed .039, or between 3 and 4 per cent., which corresponds with the percentage I have given above. This decimal would, it is true, show an excess of 39 in every thousand, but not in every hundred.

females. We have here an average deficit in favor of the females, of 9 per cent.

"How is this diversity to be explained? May it not be that woman, whose occupations are essentially sedentary, and whose habits more quiet, can accommodate herself better than man to the uniform system and routine of an asylum?"

"This supposition," continues the thoughtful writer from whom I have derived many of the figures upon which I have reasoned, "is to a certain extent justified by the small number of women who die during the first months of their admission."

Is it not more reasonable, on the other hand, in view of correlative evidence, to attribute these differences to a cause inherent in the fact of sex itself? These differences in mortality, it may, moreover, be shown, depend not merely upon varying material and economical appliances for treatment, and the varying grades of society from which patients are furnished; but they are constant. To prove this, let us compare several well-known special hospitals for either sex.

At the Bicêtre, which is exclusively for men, the mortality during the nine years from 1844 to 1852 was 263 per 1000. At the St. Lazare, which is also only for men, it was during the same period 302 per 1000; while at the Salpêtrière, which is exclusively for women, the mortality during the same period was only 177 per 1000.

At the Worcester Asylum, during its thirty-two years, there were admitted 3503 males and 3601 females, and died 426 males and 419 females; in each instance about 11 per cent. of the total admissions. From this we should at first sight surmise that the mortality of the insane was with us very much lower than it is abroad, did we not compare also the relative proportion of supposed recoveries in the two localities. If, as we have proved, these proportions do not materially vary, we have reason to suppose, if the history of our cases were carefully followed, that their mortality would not materially vary also. It is in questions like these, and more especially in those pertaining to the causation of insanity, as I may show at another time, that statistics become so unreliable. In simple inquiries like those at the commencement of this discussion, a comparison of alleged recoveries with the number of alleged admissions, for instance, there is less opportunity for error, though even here, as will soon be seen, there is abundant cause for doubt. The more complicated the question becomes, the more unreliable the result from statistics. As these have been called for, however, I desire that they should not be withheld.

In this connection, I may be pardoned for presenting some very pertinent remarks upon the subject from an authority whose loss is yet fresh to us in Massachusetts.

At the tenth annual meeting of the Association of Medical Superintendents of American Institutions for the Insane, held at Boston, in May, 1855, Dr. Bell observed that —

"He had seen no reason to change the views urged by him so many years ago in reference to the worthlessness and inexpediency of attempting to present the facts of our hospitals for the insane in a numerical form. For many years he had protested against it, both as producing unjust inferences as to different institutions, and untrue expectations in the public mind. He had labored to effect a change in this matter, and, he believed, not without success. In fact, he had rendered himself somewhat notorious, at one time, he feared, by his annual diatribe against the existing system of reporting. When visiting the most excellent institution at York, in England, 'Art thou the Luther V. Bell who has written so severely about the statistics of the insane?' was the salutation which preceded every attention and kindness which the distinguished host could give his visitor. The difficulties he feared were in the very nature of the subject. One would think that the fact of a patient being dead, for instance, was as specific, unconfoundable a basis for a statistical return as could be conceived of; yet he would engage to make his returns of dead vary fifty per cent., without one deviation from truth. A simple suggestion to friends, that it might be more agreeable to them that the last days of a failing patient should be spent in the bosom of his family, would very frequently decide whether a case of death should be on the annual return." *

At a subsequent meeting of the Association, Dr. Tyler, Dr. Bell's equally eminent successor at the McLean Asylum, took occasion to state that, though statistics might not lie, "still we know that the mor-

---

* American Journal of Insanity, xii. p. 90.

tals that make figures sometimes do." * Without in any way implying, or, indeed, believing, that this view of Dr. Tyler's is especially applicable to the point we are now considering, for the statistics that I have given were undoubtedly published in perfectly good faith by their collators, I may yet call attention to the peculiar force, in the present connection, of the last remark of Dr. Bell.

Similar comments are as applicable to the reports afforded of death details. "I do not see," says Dr. Ray, "how we can put forth as facts, of any statistical importance, the apparent causes of death. It is the custom to publish in the reports of the institution the cause of death. Now, everybody knows that in many cases this must be a matter of guess-work. I should have far less confidence in the guess of any man in regard to the cause of death in an insane person, than in one not insane." †

To return to the discussion. We may, then, justly consider, from the evidence that has been afforded, that " in those establishments which are devoted exclusively to females, the mortality, other things being equal, should be found less than in those devoted exclusively to males, the probabilities of death being, as we have already seen, greater among the latter." ‡

This fact is corroborated by Dr. Lockhart Robert-

---

* American Journal of Insanity, July, 1862, p. 44.
† Ibid., July, 1862, vol. xii. p. 38.   ‡ Legoyt, loc. cit., p. 437.

son, superintendent of the Sussex Asylum, who says that "the mean annual mortality of the male sex among the insane exceeds that of the female by about 35 per cent., while among the general population the male mortality only exceeds the female by 8 per cent." * This last excess, it will be perceived, corresponds almost exactly with the normal rate of disproportion in the sexes, which, estimated by Quetelet as averaging 106 male births alive to 100 females in Europe, has been shown by Dr. Emerson, of Philadelphia, in his excellent paper, formerly presented to this Association, to vary in this country from 107 to 110 males to 100 females.†

There is also a difference in the progressive mortality of the two sexes, according to age. Thus, from a tabular exposition of the ages at which 3303 patients deceased in the French asylums, of whom 1755 were males and 1548 females, it appears that of females at insane hospitals dying under fourteen years, there are 92 per cent. as many as men.

From 14 to 20 years,	. . .	57 per cent.
" 20 to 25 "	. . .	63 "
" 25 to 30 "	. . .	73 "
" 30 to 35 "	. . .	64 "
" 35 to 40 "	. . .	65 "
" 40 to 50 "	. . .	60 "
" 50 to 60 "	. . .	90 "

---

* Notes on the Prognosis in Mental Disease, Asylum Journal of Mental Science, January, 1859, p. 287.
† Transactions of American Medical Association, vol. iii. p. 93.

These differences are attributed by Legoyt to "the greater vitality" of the female sex. With reference to the same point, evidence concerning the relative vitality of patients considered incurable is not irrelevant.

The following table is given by Dr. Jarvis as the probable duration of life in irrecoverably insane persons. It is based upon a calculation of the expectation of life in the insane, made by the actuary of an English Life Assurance Company: — *

Age.	Males.	Females.
20	21.31 years to live.	28.66 years to live.
30	20.64 "	26.33 "
40	17.65 "	21.53 "
50	13.53 "	17.67 "
60	11.91 "	12.51 "
70	9.15 "	8.87 "

Or, in other words, the insane woman at twenty, supposed incurable, has 1.31 per cent. as many years to live as the insane man.

At 30, ...	1.23 per cent.
" 40, ...	1.07 "
" 50, ...	1.30 "
" 60, ...	1.05 "
" 70, ...	.88 "

From these facts it appears, and, as will have been seen, is acknowledged by competent authority, that —

1. The relative mortality of insane women is less than of insane men.

* Appendix to Report to Leg. of Mass., 1855, p. 192.

2. Their expectation of life, even when supposed incurable, is greater; and

3. Their percentage of recoveries, even when the mental disturbance has become chronic, is also in excess.

But how does this evidence affect the question as to whether the recoveries of women at asylums are cures?

In several ways.

In both sexes, many patients are sooner or later re-admitted to the hospital, their disease proving to have been merely palliated, not cured.

The remedial discipline to which the two sexes are subjected at asylums is almost identical. It is chiefly that which is called moral; the medical treatment in almost every instance being of a strictly general character. We are, therefore, compelled to one of two alternatives, not that more women recover at asylums than men, for this is beyond what has been claimed, or what statistics prove, but that either a certain larger proportion of insane women do not die at hospitals than men, and do recover from chronic insanity under the same general treatment, which is shown by statistical evidence, and which must arise from some primal difference in causation; or else that the character of their insanity is different, and this also implies a difference of cause, not of moral and exciting causes merely, for these on the great scale and in different countries will be found to be nearly the same, the excesses in the one instance counterbalancing all deficiencies in another, but of an intrinsic and physical character, probably sexual.

Now it will be found that those writers who deny the existence of a different physical causation of insanity in the two sexes, are no better prepared to accept the other horn of this dilemma, for it will be found that a different result from the same general treatment implies a difference in disease; and a difference in disease arising from the excitement of similar stimuli, implies a difference in predisposition, and therefore, in ultimate causation.

The only escape from these conclusions, is by denying my premises as to the character and identity of the medical treatment resorted to for the two sexes. Upon this point, however, though I have already furnished sufficient evidence, I will add still more.

Again, most writers on insanity acknowledge a frequent influence of the catamenia and of the catamenial molimen in reference to the exacerbation of the mental disturbance; this, to a certain extent, putting aside the question as to whether or no the insanity in any of these cases springs from a uterine origin. To the extent now stated, few will deny the fact, for an immense body of proof has been incidentally published in psychological text books, monographs, and periodicals, and can be readily adduced.

In many of these cases, the menses when absent have *accidentally* appeared without any direct aid from medical treatment, and the patient has immediately and in consequence recovered. Such cases are not spoken of as uncommon. They undoubtedly frequently occur.

Many instances are also on record, where insanity has suddenly ceased on the woman's passing the grand climacteric, at the permanent and final cessation of the catamenia. It could hardly be alleged that these were cases of *cure*. They also, there is good reason to believe, are not uncommon.

It will be seen that I here purposely avoid referring to other than published and acknowledged evidence furnished by the directors of asylums, for almost every work as yet issued upon the subject of insanity has been from such a source.

There is one other point to which, in this connection, I may be permitted to refer, and that, the comparative infrequency in women of one of the most common and most fatal of the forms of insanity. I refer to the so-called paralysis of the insane, the paralysie générale of the usual and artificial classification.

This disease, one of the few mental disorders that is attended by organic lesion of the brain, or rather of the medulla oblongata and spinal cord, is comparatively unknown in women. This fact has been acknowledged by Dr. Robertson, of the Sussex Asylum,* by Drs. Workman and Choate† in this country, and by many other competent authorities. "We know positively," says Morel, "that the number of the (general) paralytic insane is infinitely greater among men than among women." ‡

In a table furnished by the author now quoted, it appears that of 800 insane women at the asylum of St. Yon, there were 25 afflicted with this disease, or 3 per cent.; while at the asylum of Quatre Mares, devoted exclusively to males, there were of 500 inmates no less than 100, or 20 per cent., affected with general paralysis.

It is undoubtedly this disease that was referred to by Esquirol, when he says, —

"Paralysis is more frequent among insane men than women. Eighteen years ago, when charged with the service of the division of the insane at the Bicêtre, during the absence of M. Pariset, who was sent to Cadiz to study the yellow fever which was prevailing there, I was struck, in comparing the number of men, insane and paralytic, at the Bicêtre, and the number of paralytic women at the Salpêtrière. The same observation may be made in every establishment into which both sexes are admitted. It has not escaped the notice of Dr. Foville, physician-in-chief at St. Yon. According to this physician, they amount to one eleventh at the institution over which he presides. Among 334 insane persons who were examined by him, 31 were paralytic, to wit, 22 men and 9 women. At Charenton, the proportion of paralytics is still more considerable. They constitute one sixth of the whole number of admissions. In

---

* Asylum Journal of Mental Science, January, 1859, p. 276.
† American Journal of Insanity, 1860.
‡ Traité des Maladies Mentales, p. 813.

truth, of 619 insane persons who were admitted during the three years, 1826, 1827, and 1828, 109 were paralytics. But the proportion of men is enormous compared with that of women. Of 366 insane men admitted into the house, 95 were paralytics; while of 153 women, 14 only were affected with paralysis. This complication is most frequently observed among that class of insane persons who have yielded to venereal excesses, or have been addicted to the use of alcoholic drinks; among those, also, who have made an inordinate use of mercury, as well as those who, exercising the brain too vigorously in mental strife, have at the same time abandoned themselves to errors of regimen. Do not these circumstances explain sufficiently well how it happens that there are more men insane and paralytic than women?"*

The few cases of women who are affected by general paralysis are chiefly prostitutes,† so that in the ordinary classes of society, it is among women practically absent. The fact to which I have referred is one that is now generally acknowledged. In a discussion upon the subject at Philadelphia, in 1860, it was fully admitted by Drs. Workman of Toronto, Bancroft of the New Hampshire State Asylum, Athon of that of Indiana, and Harlow of that of Maine.‡

The same comparative immunity for women has also been noted in the form of insanity now known as congestive mania, and so thoroughly described by my colleague, Dr. Worthington, of the Friends' Asylum at Frankford, Pa.§

* Esquirol, loc. cit., p. 438.
† Morel: Traités des Maladies Mentales, p. 828.
‡ American Journal of Insanity, July, 1860, p. 65.
§ Ibid., p. 64. — October, 1850, p. 114.

We may, from the evidence that has now been offered, fairly conclude, that (1) while some at least of the women discharged from asylums as recovered, are not in reality cases of cure, (2) there are others not reported as having recovered, who yet ought, if we may believe the evidence of statistics, to have done so. If the mortality in insane women is less than in men, and if the most frequent of the incurable mental diseases in men is absent in women, a larger percentage of them should recover than of men, unless they have some corresponding fatal disease which is absent in men. The existence however of such a disease has never been acknowledged.

If the facts above proved are admitted, it would seem (3) that all justifiable resources of medical treatment can scarcely have been put in requisition at asylums.

I have alluded, in connection with the last point now referred to, to the admissions of gentlemen having asylums in charge. In a former communication upon this subject, I stated why it was that, as asylums are now constituted, the whole duty of a physician by his patient, if a woman, could not be performed.* The evidence was such as was thought conclusive by the American Medical Association, at its late meeting in New York. That there might be no room for cavil, I fortified my arguments by a frank and forcible letter

---

* Boston Medical and Surgical Journal, October, 1864, p. 211.

from Dr. Butler, of the Hartford Retreat.* The force of this letter was subsequently sought to be weakened, by the assertion "that it was only conclusive of the lack of a disposition on the part of its writer to make use of all the means of treatment considered proper to aid in restoring a patient." † That the position of Dr. Butler, as described by himself, is a very common one, I have good reason to believe; and as it arises from causes over which superintendents have had no control, I have not been so unjust as to throw any blame upon them, as their own official brother seems to have done in the communication to which I have referred.

The same charge of incompetence, implied if not directly made, against these gentlemen, has come to me from another quarter of their own precincts. Under date of 11th January, 1865, Dr. Gray, of the New York State Lunatic Asylum at Utica, writes me as follows: —

"Of the applicability of some of your strictures to some asylum superintendents,‡ it is not for me to judge. I, however, contend that they do not apply to all, any more than would a sweeping charge of ignorance against the medical faculty of Harvard, on account of the incapacity of some of your professional brethren." §

---

* Boston Medical and Surgical Journal, October, 1864, p. 214.
† Ibid., November, 1864, p. 290.
‡ It will have been noticed by those familiar with my former papers, that my strictures were upon no asylum superintendents, but upon the circumstances which prevent their performing their whole duty by their patients.
§ Had Dr. Gray the gift of prophecy? might now, in 1870, well be asked.

I can only say, in reference to this point, that the only instances in which evidence has been furnished me that what is generally styled special treatment for the diseases peculiar to women, such as is now constantly resorted to, and generally considered proper and necessary in civil practice, has ever been employed at any of our insane asylums, save at the Butler Hospital, at Providence, and at the McLean Asylum, in consultation, have been at the Friends' Hospital, at Frankford, Pa., and at the Michigan State Asylum, at Kalamazoo, respectively under the charge of my colleagues, Drs. Worthington and Van Deusen. I may in this matter do great injustice to the zeal of those eminent in this specialty, and to their moral courage, for this is needed in instituting what I have proved to be a radical change in treatment, but, as I have made minute inquiries, and have now heard from many of the gentlemen referred to, it is hardly possible.

In the case of the Utica Asylum, from which one of the implications alluded to has come, I can only say that this is one of quite a number of asylums that I have had opportunity, officially, carefully to examine; that my visit to it was in September, 1863; that in the absence of Dr. Gray, the superintendent, I was most courteously received by his very intelligent assistant physicians, who freely and fully informed me concerning all points that I raised, which were chiefly with reference to the medical treatment of the female patients; that from what I was told, I have no reason to suppose that special treatment was thought necessary at that asylum for the so common special diseases of women, whether occurring as cause of the insanity, or its concomitant; and that I had very good reason, on the contrary, to believe that such was seldom or never resorted to at the present time.* If, however, I was mistaken in my impression, — and I shall be most happy to learn that I was in error, — then it will follow that Dr. Gray himself, and all gentlemen who are sufficiently enlightened to engage in the investigations for which I am contending, and which, from the language I have quoted, he would seem to approve, it will follow that they all, equally with myself, fall under the ban laid in the Boston Medical and Surgical Journal for 5th January, 1865, upon every one of us who would cure in insane women their so-called "imaginary" physical disease; † as supposed to be present, not by them, but by ourselves.

I have said that my remarks do not apply to our own asylums alone, nor have I desired that they

---

* Yet in the report of the New York State Asylum for 1852, by Dr. Gray, it appears that in nearly one fourth of all the cases of insanity reported, the disturbance of the generative organs was so marked as to be regarded as a *primary* cause of the mental derangement. (Amer. Journal of Insanity, xii. p. 306.) In the report of the same institution ten years later, for 1862, only a tenth of the women are thus reported, unless the forty-three cases stated as caused by previous ill health are to be considered of this character, in which event, the proportion would rise to nearly one half.

† Loc. cit., pp. 452 and 453.

should seem to do so. The similarity as to percentages of recoveries, &c., between our own and foreign asylums, goes to prove what I have attempted to show by other evidence, that nowhere, at home or abroad, has the difference of causation which, I believe, exists in many instances between the two sexes as to mental disease, been generally appreciated or acted upon. The view to which I refer explains the problems elicited by the statistics I have now presented; they, on the other hand, are wholly inexplicable, save by this simple key. I may be told over and over again that my view is an old one. If appreciated in all its bearings, why then has it not been accepted? That it has been so in the present, or in former times, I can find no evidence.

The disturbance which my deductions seem to have caused in certain minds, would seem to imply, as I have indeed been told, that there was a chance that these inquiries, if pushed, would result in injury to the present unimpeded system of hospital management. Nothing, however, as I have already asserted in almost every paper I have written upon the subject, is further from my own intention. The researches have been undertaken simply and solely for a scientific purpose, and the papers I have now presented may serve as earnest that the investigations will be pushed to their legitimate result, it is almost unnecessary to state, without either fear or favor.

It was lately publicly intimated, that for one of the measures I have advocated, merely one item in the system of public and private treatment that is required for insane women, the establishment of an Advisory Medical Board at asylums,* there can be found no one of any note among superintendents to approve. I will not weary my readers by carrying my evidence from statistics to any greater extent than I have already done, though I am well prepared even upon this point. I will, therefore, simply append the following letter, which was unsolicited, from Dr. Isaac Ray:—

"BUTLER HOSPITAL, Nov. 26, 1864.

"MY DEAR SIR: I have read your pamphlet with much interest, especially your remarks on the employment of Boards of Consulting Physicians in asylums for the insane. Your views strike me to be eminently just, and I am glad you have called public attention to the subject. The case, in fact, hardly admits of argument. What medical man now needs be persuaded that in a hospital of at least one hundred patients, for any disease, there must be occasions, more or less, when the single doctor in charge would or should gladly consult another physician? And if so, it is

---

* Trans. Amer. Med. Association, 1864. With regard to the suggestion now referred to, I would frankly state that my colleagues, Drs. Van Deusen and Worthington, like some others of the fraternity who have erroneously seen in the advisory board an end rather than a means, are disinclined to indorse it; basing their objections, so far as communicated to me, upon the trite ground that any assistance would be rather an interference with the superintendents. The former of the gentlemen, however, admits that "the subject of the appointment of a consulting physician and surgeon, *with special* reference to the examination and surgical treatment of female patients requiring it, is new" to him; and it is allowed by the latter that "there might be cases, here and there, that would (thus) be helped."

far better that he should resort to an established Board, made expressly for his benefit, ready to come gratuitously, than to some eminent man who expects and is justly entitled to a liberal compensation. To such a Board as I refer, the honor of the position would always be considered sufficient compensation for so light a duty.

"Your paper seems to be but part of a larger one, which, if published, I have not been so fortunate as to meet. Unquestionably, abnormal conditions of the sexual organs have often a very large influence in the development of insanity in women. I presume, however, my observations would hardly warrant me in attributing so much to them as, I suppose, from one or two expressions, you do.

"I admit that we asylum physicians cannot, necessarily, obtain that accuracy of diagnosis which is comparatively easy to other men; but the existence of sexual disorder of some kind need not be overlooked by any one who looks at all, provided it is sufficiently grave to affect the brain.* Not that I consider these affections as of little consequence, and unworthy, when present, of being accurately understood and properly treated, for I am well aware that mental disease may sometimes be continued indefinitely by the persistent influence of sexual organic disorder.

"We had here this summer a death in the earlier stage of mania, where the disease seemed to have been mainly excited by some venereal excrescences in the vagina, and we have now in the house a lady whose disease was unquestionably produced, as it is now kept up, by an 'irritable uterus.'

"I repeat that I am glad you have called attention to this point, because, in the treatment of insanity, we are too apt to overlook or undervalue all collateral, subordinate conditions.

"Yours, very respectfully,
"I. RAY.
"Dr. H. R. Storer."

---

* Dr. Ray seems here hardly to appreciate the nice discriminations, so often productive of success in treatment, now made in the diagnosis, direct and differential, of pelvic disease.

The following is the Report above alluded to: —

"In late communications to the American Academy of Arts and Sciences, and to the Suffolk District Medical Society of Massachusetts,* I have stated certain fundamental propositions or laws, whose acceptance is essential to any rational explanation or treatment of the mental diseases of women. These propositions are as follows: —

"I. That in women mental disease is often, perhaps generally, dependent upon functional or organic disturbance of the reproductive system.

"II. That in women the access or exacerbation of mental disease is usually coincident with the catamenial establishment, its periodical access, or final cessation.

"III. That the rational and successful treatment of mental disease in women must be based upon the preceding theories, which I claim are established, —

"1. By many analogies, physiological and pathological, in the cerebral manifestations of the human female and of the lower mammals;

"2. By clinical observation; and

"3. By the results of autopsies of the insane, both in private practice and, where made with equal impartiality, in insane asylums.

"I have worded the last expression with especial reference to the facts, that in autopsies by psychological specialists diseases of the brain are naturally those first sought for; and that in autopsies of insane women, as compared with those of insane men, disease of the brain, as a primary lesion, very rarely exists. These facts are acknowledged; for further remarks upon them I must refer to the preliminary paper to which I have already alluded.

"From the above propositions, corroborated, I believe, by the experience of every unbiassed observer, we advance to three plain and practical questions, which are to open up

---

* Boston Medical and Surgical Journal, April, 1864. p. 189.

a new, broad, and very fruitful field of gynæcological work
These are, —

"1. To what extent can the insanity of women be medically or surgically treated?

"2. Is such treatment at present generally effected, or even attempted, in insane hospitals? and, —

"3. How can it there be accomplished?

"I am aware that I have broached a delicate topic. The comparison, however, of doubtfully insane, of almost insane, and of decidedly insane women, in all their range, from aggravated hysteria to actual madness, has so long been my daily occupation that I am enabled to express myself plainly upon this subject. It is one that has been hitherto neglected, for the sole reason that its proper side of approach — that from a gynæcological point — happens, from circumstances beyond their control, almost always to have been closed to superintendents and others charged with the management of the insane.

"The first question that I have now proposed, To what extent can the insanity of women be medically and surgically treated? has as yet hardly been propounded in insane asylums at all, although its solution in active, everyday practice is, within certain limits, of common enough occurrence. I have purposely limited my statement of the extent to which this treatment has as yet been carried in private practice. Instances in point, however, — the ordinary forms of the so-called puerperal mania, and of that other type of insanity to which in its different manifestations I would attach the equally legitimate title of catamenial mania, — are familiar to every observer. In these and in others of the host of deviations from mental sanity in women, there is some reflex transferrence of irritative action, the source of which, if searched for, is almost always to be discovered. It is just as unscientific here, and generally as futile, to treat merely or primarily the mental disturbance, which is usually a symptom only or a consequence, as it has been to amputate an hysterical knee, to attempt the Cæsarean section or to cut for ovariotomy in cases of the so-called spurious pregnancy, or, as is still constantly done, even at the present day, to stimulate or blister, or apply the moxa or actual cautery to spines irritated sympathetically and through reflex action by an abraded, displaced, or otherwise disturbed womb. The necessity of removing a cause, to prevent or to cure its effect, is as decided in mental pathology as in physical. We recognize it everywhere else; we must recognize it in the treatment of insane women, no matter whether, from quiet and inoffensive creatures, or chaste and pure, they have become habitually thievish, profane, or obscene, despondent or self-indulgent, shrewish or fatuous, or, as the parturient cat or sow, they have destroyed their offspring, or, in other cases, have attempted to destroy themselves.

"In many of these instances, the relation of cause to effect, if otherwise doubtful, is at once shown by the result of the treatment. I might relate many cases in illustration of this fact from my own experience, but shall confine myself to a single one.

"*Case.* During the past year I have had charge of a young lady afflicted with that not uncommon disease, mechanical dysmenorrhœa. This patient, unmarried, and formerly a school-teacher, was sent to me by a physician, and had previously consulted several others. She confessed to me that while she never had had sexual intercourse, she had experienced, from a period long preceding her first seeking medical aid, excessive sexual desire, amounting, indeed, to what is technically termed nymphomania — a symptom merely, as are most of the mental disturbances of women. The attacks of this were very clearly coincident with the menstrual period, and so extreme that the patient could with difficulty restrain herself from soliciting the approach of the other sex. She could not restrain herself from frequent and excessive masturbation. There was little irritability about the clitoris or other external organs, the patient herself being inclined to recognize a deeper and inner origin for her suffering. The morbid desires, and the disgusting propensity thence arising, ceased together with the dysmenorrhœal pain, upon freely incising the cervix uteri, and dilating its canal. They have not since returned, save in one single instance, when an acute attack of the erotic desire, plainly resulting from indulgence in so-called pepper tea, was at once allayed by the application of potassa fusa to the cervix. Now, were not this treatment based, as it is, upon a broad and general physiological principle, its effect as a defence, in similar cases, to female chastity, threatened and undermined by sources of irritation within the patient herself, would be sufficient to entitle it to our respectful consideration. The above case must not be thought more pertinent than others of a similar reflex character, where, however, there is no erotic desire or other direct symptom of genital irritation. However masked, they all instance a single law.

" It would be difficult to state precisely to what extent appropriate medical and surgical treatment can be effectual in the cure of female insanity, the subject as presented in this light being comparatively new to the profession. There can be little doubt, however, that in so far as the mental disturbance retains its original reflex character, and has not merged into organic cerebral change, which, as I have said, is comparatively rare in women, to this extent and so long should we have a reasonable hope of success, nearly as great, perhaps, as in relieving the other reflex disturbances to which the female is confessedly so prone.

" As regards the second question I have broached, Is such treatment effected, or even attempted, in insane hospitals? the answer is patent. As hospitals are at present organized, the proper treatment cannot be afforded insane women, for sufficient reason.

" To the general organization of our public asylums, or to its details, so far as they go, I would take no exception. My complaint is, that their most excellent organizations do not go quite far enough to cover the important class of cases we are now considering. They stop just one step short of the mark. I am here speaking from personal observation of the working, theoretical and practical, of many asylums, among the best in this country — and there are in the world none in advance of the American hospitals for the insane;

so that in my remarks upon this subject I speak with perfect confidence.

"The reason that mental disease in the female, dependent upon reflex uterine or ovarian irritation, is not generally treated at hospitals for the insane in the same manner, or as successfully, barring only the lessened risk of homicide or of suicide before cure, as in private practice, is in the main the following: —

"The whole and sole charge of the patients, medical, moral, and economical, is thrown entirely upon the superintendent of the hospital. This is certainly an advantage in everything concerning the government of the establishment, for it prevents all clash of opinion, all evasions of duty. It is excellent in every respect, save alone as concerns the weight and the extent of medical responsibility. I would by no means lessen the superintendent's authority, but, as will be seen, would free him from his present involuntary embarrassment.

"The superintendent, as at present situated, cannot make such examination of a female patient, or pursue such methods of treatment, as are absolutely required for the relief of many forms of gynæcological disease, upon the existence of which, as I have said, her mental malady not unfrequently depends. He is absolutely prevented from this alike by regard for the patient's welfare, for his own personal reputation, and for that of his hospital. So constantly compelled to see the patient, he appreciates the importance, as regards other details of treatment, moral, etc., that he should retain her confidence and escape her fears; he recognizes the danger lest an endeavor to arrive at a proper diagnosis of her disease should seem to the disordered mind only an attempt at improper and unpardonable liberties with her person, and should she ever entirely recover her reason, be so represented to friends and to the community by her perverted and imperfect memory. These risks, so great in sane patients under temporary aberration from anæsthesia, have been realized to the full by Dr. Beale, of Philadelphia, and others; with the insane they are increased.

"In this strait, upon whom is the superintendent to rely? Not upon his assistants, surely — younger men, and often merely pupils, at any rate placed in the same relations as himself to the patient, the hospital, and the outside world. Here is the strange and paradoxical example of a physician pledged by even higher than ordinary motives to the relief of his suffering patients, concerning a large proportion of whom, however, his hands and his judgment are practically and entirely fettered. He cannot search for the manifestations of disease, nor, were they known to be present, can he relieve them; and yet we all contend, and strive to persuade the community, that our hospitals for the insane are no longer prisons; that they are not houses for detention, but for cure. The existence of these facts, and the justness of the above reasoning, superintendents have repeatedly acknowledged to me with regret, and a hope that the evil may be remedied.

"A change is necessary: how can it be accomplished? By appointing to every asylum in the land a board of consulting physicians — useful in ordinary cases of insanity, but absolutely indispensable in the instance of insane women. These gentlemen should be selected from practitioners in the immediate neighborhood of each asylum, due regard, of course, being had to their character and to their professional fitness. The position should be an honorary one, and, like that at general hospitals, unattended by pecuniary emolument; and the superintendent should be left entirely to use his own discretion as to calling or not upon the members of his board for advice, just as is allowed to attending physicians or surgeons at general hospitals, the intention being to render consultations and a division of medical responsibility possible, not compulsory. Strange as it may seem, there appears to exist but a single asylum in this country to which there is appended a board of medical consultation. I refer to that most admirable establishment, the Butler Hospital, at Providence. So far as I have been able to ascertain, — and I have been aided by those most excellent authorities in all matters pertaining to the insane, Drs.

Ray, of Rhode Island, and Edward Jarvis, of Massachusetts, — in no instance, save the one referred to, have boards of medical advice been included among their officers and means of management at our insane hospitals.

"The Connecticut Retreat has a Board of Medical Visitors, whose position is an anomalous one: as much supervisors of general administration, apparently, as advisory in the treatment of patients, they are, perhaps, in reality, more strictly honorary than either.

"There was formerly an Advisory Board attached to the City Lunatic Hospital of New York, at Blackwell's Island, discontinued for no known reason.

"The New York Hospital has Consulting Surgeons and Consulting Physicians; but they appear to have nothing to do with the Bloomingdale Asylum, although it is under the same general authority as the hospital. The case is similar to that of the McLean Asylum, which, though under the same trustees, is yet separate from the Massachusetts General Hospital. The last has Consulting Physicians and Surgeons, but they have nothing to do with the insane department. They may, it is true, have been occasionally consulted by Dr. Bell, and possibly by his successors, in cases of doubtful sickness of a general character, just as other gentlemen, from time to time, have been called upon to give opinion. As matters now remain, such consultations are wholly unofficial, and Dr. Ray's establishment, therefore, would seem at present to stand alone, and to furnish, with its skilful advisory staff of Drs. Mauran and Miller, an example to be followed.

"So far these remarks have been based upon my own personal observation of the needs and advantages of the measure I have proposed. I am able to go farther than this, however, and to give corroborative evidence from superintendents themselves.

"In a report recently rendered to the Legislature of Massachusetts, the views of the writer as one of the State Commissioners in Insanity were embodied, he fully recognizing, however, and admitting the fact that the appointment of boards of medical consultation, as a part of the internal management of hospitals, should devolve upon their boards of trustees, and in no way be controlled by the State. The various opinions and recommendations presented in the report alluded to were very properly submitted to the Superintendents of the several State asylums by the Legislative Committee to which it had been referred, and almost without exception they were cordially indorsed. With respect to the propriety of appointing consulting physicians to the hospitals there was not a dissenting voice; Drs. Tyler, of the McLean Asylum, Walker, of that at South Boston, and Choate, of the Taunton Hospital, acknowledging that they had each felt the need of such assistance, and would gladly avail themselves of it were it afforded them, while Dr. Ray, of Providence, who alone could speak from personal experience of its advantages, gave the Committee to understand that he considered his Board as at once comfort, relief, and safeguard. Such would probably be found to be the unanimous opinion of gentlemen engaged in this most responsible specialty.

"I have now presented the subject only in its relations to patient and superintendent, and have endeavored to show the advantages and necessity, alike to both, of the measure proposed. I might well cease here, confident that my remarks have been sufficiently conclusive. The subject is no less important, however, to the community at large, in its relations to gynæcological practice and obstetric jurisprudence.

"Gynæcological practice, as I have already hinted, covers legitimately the greater number of cases of female insanity, but it is to hospitals for the insane that the profession must necessarily send many of these patients, and it is to hospitals for the insane that we must therefore look for the most effectual trial of rational methods of treatment, and from them trust for examples of successful cure. For this success they have already, with the single exception alluded to, every possible adjunct: seclusion of their patients from exciting causes; their absolute control as to diet, habits, and whole detail of life; the possibility, so far as skilled attendance is concerned, of carrying out any desired plan of treatment. Were such indorsed by men experienced in similar methods as applied in every-day practice, the superintendent's responsibilities, doubts, and risks would all be lightened, and the measures indicated be readily enough pursued. Before long there would be a mass of digested observations and medical reports issuing from these very hospitals, which would be of immense value to the profession in civil life.

"I have referred, and I trust it will not be thought with disrespect, to the tendencies at asylums, in the search for cerebral lesion, to ignore all others. I could relate many instances corroborative of this fact, but it is unnecessary. The very nature of mental disturbance would of itself be sufficient to explain it, did we not have additional reason in the position in which I have shown hospital officers to stand in relation to their cases of insane women. It is evident in the very details of asylum autopsies as compared with those at general hospitals, in the statements of appearances found, and in the silence upon points not supposed essential. I would not imply that there are not most faithful and thorough pathologists among psychologists—a combination, of which Dr. Workman, of Toronto, is by far the most excellent example with whom I am personally acquainted; nor do I believe there are many superintendents in this country who sympathize with their other Canadian representative, Dr. Douglass, of the Lower Province, whose assertion to me of contemptuous disbelief in the need or advantage of autopsies of the insane, was only additional proof, had such been needed, that his Government Asylum at Beaufort, near Quebec, however fair in outside seeming, is based on an erroneous view of management; that it is conducted for private rather than for public good, and, by comparison with that of Canada West, that it should be abated as an error and a nuisance by Parliament.* This is no digression.

* This was in 1864. I am informed (1870) that the suggestion above made was effectual in producing the necessary change.

The topic, both personal and theoretical, is one intimately related to that we have been considering, and I shall discuss it more fully upon another occasion. When autopsies of insane females shall have become more frequent and more carefully studied, the importance of the doctrines now urged will become the more apparent.

"I have intimated that the appointment of medical advisers to insane hospitals would be of advantage to obstetric jurisprudence.

"We are all familiar with those difficult cases of supposed or alleged insanity in females that from time to time make their appearance in our courts of justice, on writs of *habeas corpus* or otherwise, from asylums, puzzling counsel, medical experts, and judge. Such cases are common enough in private practice, and are found generally amenable to treatment. There is no reason that they should still be allowed to serve as excitants of public scandal, or to bring discredit upon hospital management, or to subject their officers to suspicion as venal.

"There is a vast field above and beyond all this, which many writers have approached, none more boldly than lately Dr. Ray* — important beyond all estimate in its jurisprudential relations, but which has hardly as yet been entered, certainly not to any extent, from the quarter in which we are now standing. I refer to the legal and moral responsibilities of women, whether maniacal or but partially affected; a matter of infinite interest, of infinite practical importance, I can now but allude to it. It is another proof to us of what may be the results, scientific and effective, from insane asylums when they shall have been made what they may more fully become, hospitals for research, for rational experiment, and for cure.

"In accordance with the arguments now submitted, I would offer the following resolutions, which I trust the Association may unanimously see reason, in its wisdom, to adopt and to render effective: —

---

* Treatise on Mental Hygiene; Report of Butler Hospital for 1864.

"*Resolved*, That in the opinion of the American Medical Association it is expedient that there should be attached to every public hospital for the insane, one or more consulting physicians, who may be consulted at the discretion of the superintendent; such measure being alike for the interest of the hospital, its medical officers, and its patients.

"*Resolved*, That a copy of the above resolution be transmitted to the Board of Trustees of each of our public hospitals for the insane; and also to the Secretary of the Association of American Superintendents, with the request that it may be indorsed by that body, and the action proposed be urged upon the respective boards with which its members are officially connected." *

I have thus, very imperfectly as I am aware, presented a portion of my views as to the causation and treatment of a large proportion of the cases of insanity occurring in women. I have furnished evidence, in confirmation of these views, from many of the leading psychological experts of the present day. I have shown that my deductions are such as *à priori* ought to have resulted, and such as alone can explain admitted facts. I have proved that these views are not generally entertained by the specialty devoted to the insane, or if entertained, are not generally acted upon in practice. I have confined myself in the main to the general question of causation, for the present omitting the discussion of minor but scarcely less important questions and details; upon all of which I have now a mass of evidence, that I shall hereafter

---

* The above paper having been read before the Section on Obstetrics, and warmly approved by many of its members, the resolutions appended were referred to the Association at large, and were indorsed by a unanimous vote.

most gladly adduce. I have refrained, save in what pertains to pregnancy, from using the testimony of gynæcologists, and of the profession at large, strongly corroborative as this would have been of my every position, preferring to meet the objections that have been made, by answers from a similar source. I have attempted to avoid all resort, or appearance of resort, to any special pleading, though such is apparent enough in these objections; that, for instance, a gynæcologist must necessarily be a practitioner of but one idea, and therefore incompetent — the truth being, that without at least one fundamental idea, no man should be deemed fit for the charge of any sick women, whether insane or in their right mind.

I have endeavored to deal fairly with gentlemen whose opinions, from a previous bias of perhaps many years' standing, may clash with my own, and have acknowledged my belief that, in most of the quarters of this important sphere, they have left little unaccomplished that was practicable for the good of their patients. I have striven sedulously to avoid expressions or a tone that could possibly create undue offence — though not, I conceive, upon all occasions, myself treated as fairly. With reference to certain of the arguments with which I have been met, I might well have said, as did Blundell in answering the current criticisms upon ovariotomy, for our cases are in many respects very parallel: "These men are butting their heads against a stone wall; and the grimaces they make, on feeling the solidity of the materials, are as amusing as they are pitiable." Had I not, at this time at least, decided to fortify my plea by evidence that had been afforded solely by psychologists, I might have adduced more trenchant commentaries than I have done, even indeed from the authorities I have made use of.

But, on the other hand, it is a good rule in medicine that where there is a choice of measures, the harshest is always to be chosen the last. It is as true of the birth of a principle or of a method of practice, as of a child. In surgery, no incision is to be made longer or deeper than the occasion requires. Sincerely believing, as I do, that the only rational treatment of insane women must be based upon the same general medical and surgical principles as those that control the management of every other conceivable form of disease, I could say no less than I have done. To the profession I leave the decision of the questions involved.

A few days subsequently to the meeting of the Association at which the above report was presented, I attended, as its delegate, the Annual Meeting at Pittsburg of the Association of American Superintendents, with instructions to urge upon these gentlemen the propriety, for the purposes of science and of effectual practice, of a more intimate union upon their part with our own body, representing as this does the profession at large. The cordiality with which I was received by the large circle of Superintendents then present, the majority of them till then strangers to me, and the respectful attention with which my views, so far as I presented them, were met, have but served to confirm me in the opinion that those who have so ungraciously endeavored to stifle this discussion do not represent the main body of American psychologists, and that the seeds of a more rational practice, now to be scattered by the aid of the press, will not fall upon wholly unfruitful soil.

The following is the report which was rendered to the American Medical Association at its meeting the ensuing year, 1866.

"At the last meeting of this Association the undersigned was appointed its delegate to the Association of Medical Superintendents of American Institutions for the Insane, for the purpose of urging upon that body the advantages of a more intimate union with your own, alike for the purposes of science and effectual practice. Having attended to the duty confided to him, he would render the following report: —

"Four days after your own adjournment, your delegate met the associated superintendents at Pittsburg, Pa., and communicated to them your expressed desire, urging, at the same time, the mutual advantage that would ensue to both parties interested, themselves and yourselves, from the action proposed. He was very courteously received and hospitably entertained by the Association of Superintendents, and your request was listened to with the respect that its importance demanded, many gentlemen seeming alive to the necessity that the proposed union should be effected.

When, however, the question was taken, your proposal was not acceded to, and a different time and place than your own were fixed for the meeting of the superintendents the present year.

"By his action in the premises, your delegate might seem relieved from further remark. Having discussed this matter, however, as he has done, with the gentlemen comprising the offstanding association, and become familiar with their temper and opinions upon this very important subject, he would have but half fulfilled his duty did he refrain from expressing his views concerning the present position. He does this the more cheerfully, from the fact that the recent meeting of the superintendents at Washington, though not held in accordance with your desire, has permitted a larger number of superintendents than usual to attend your own convocation; and though, by their action, it has been rendered impossible for you to send a delegate to their meeting of the present year, as you decided by vote to continue to do until the proposed union shall have been effected, the opportunity has been afforded for you to reiterate your opinion, not through a delegate merely, but in your own persons, as now assembled.

"The views referred to naturally subdivide themselves according as they relate — 1st, to the welfare of this Association; 2dly, to that of the profession at large; 3dly, to that of the great class of sick persons more directly interested in your action, namely, the insane; 4thly, to that of the community; and it might be added, 5thly, to that of the superintendents of asylums themselves.

"1. Of what advantage is it to this Association that it represent, in reality, the profession of the country? It would, at first sight, seem that this question could hardly have been soberly asked, its answer is so very evident; and yet, practically, its discussion at the present moment and in the present connection is well worthy your attention. In this brief report, however, there can be offered but a very few words.

"That a house divided against itself cannot stand, is as

true in your affairs as in those of other men. The position of the Association of Superintendents towards your own organization is unlike that of the ordinary medical bodies represented in your councils by delegates. It is itself a great centralizing power, effectual, to a certain extent, no doubt, for good; effectual also for harm. Its conferences have been the means of eliciting an immense deal of important information concerning the hygienic management and economic detail of asylums; which could, however, with equal, and indeed greater, advantage have been presented through your own channel. On the other hand, these communications have not been presented directly to the profession; few of whom, indeed, do they reach at all. The Association of Superintendents and its official publication — the one composed of, and the other conducted by, however competent men — constitute, in reality, a partition wall between the very important department of the profession they represent and your own great body of workers, the profession at large.

"In all specialties — and the care of the insane is but such — the practitioner has little reason to separate himself from his fellows. He is incompetent for his work unless he has himself been tried in the furnace of general practice; he is unfit for it if he is unwilling to freely communicate with the mass of his profession. Researches merely for the benefit of a limited circle, publications merely for a few selected readers, alike fail of the two great ends that alone should be sought by the true physician — the general edification of his professional brethren, and the general relief of those sick persons whom he professes to wish to cure.

"Viewed in this light, the profession and this Association, its representative, have a right to claim, from every one of its members, individual and combined efforts for the general good; and, looking upon separate and close organizations with a certain measure of very natural distrust, it is clearly your duty to use such measures as may afford themselves to claim for this body a more hearty allegiance.

"However decided one's sympathy with efforts to advance

all legitimate specialties, still the good of the general practitioner must rise superior to all other considerations. For this reason, every attempt to directly separate any class of specialists from the mass of their fellows is to be deprecated. The ophthalmologists of this country, for instance, who comprise among their number some of your most worthy brethren, are doing much for the glory of medicine; yet it is to be lamented that they should desire, by organizing themselves into a separate Association, practically to dissociate their department from its legitimate and influential connection with the parent body, as one of its chief and strongest supports.

"Through your so-called Sections, wisely and, if thought necessary, permanently organized, all the work of special organizations can be effected as thoroughly as by any other method, and with infinitely more advantage to the mass of the profession.

"2. Whatever redounds to the advantage of this Association, either as regards the respect and honor in which it is held or the influence it is enabled to exert, is necessarily also to the advantage of its individual members, and the institutions, whether hospitals, societies, or schools, that they represent. This body should be considered, as was the aim of its founders, the exponent of American medical position and scientific acquirement. That the possibility of this actually taking place has been in some quarters inconsiderately made light of, is neither proof nor argument that it cannot be effected. Selection you have from all worth the culling. It only requires a wise combination of forces to render these, your forces, effective powers — effective to raise the standard of medical education, practice, and result. You cannot afford to allow any of your main departments to attempt an independent crusade. In union alone is there the completest strength, and the strength of the whole is in reality the strength of each individual of your numbers from the profession at large.

"3. There can be no doubt as to the advantage to the great class of the insane, of a more direct and personal interest in their welfare on the part of physicians generally, than now obtains. Were it absolutely certain that there could be no possible advance in the knowledge and treatment of insanity, the case might be different; but the experience of the past with all its great changes, most of them reforms, teaches otherwise. That our asylums are so excellently managed, officered by such competent superintendents, and fruitful to the extent they are of improvement in their patients, affords undoubted cause for laudation; but this is a very different thing from being perfect. The mere fact that so large a proportion of insane patients has thus far proved incurable is surely a reason for bending to the subject the scrutiny of a larger and larger number of skilled investigators, and so perhaps eventually working for the insane of the present day as great a revolution in respect to improvement as was effected by Pinel for those of the past. As one most efficient agent towards such increased interest in the study of insanity would be found a closer union of superintendents with your own Association.

"4. To the community there would be gains, over and above these already enumerated, were the Association reënforced by those gentlemen who have practically seceded from its ranks. There exists still too prevalently the feeling that asylums for the insane are in reality but prisons, under a less repulsive name. It is needless to deny the fact. Every physician is aware of the impression to which reference is now made, and of the check it exerts in many unhappy instances upon the needed transferrence of a patient to a more suitable and healthful mental atmosphere.

"Now asylums should be stripped of this odium still clinging to them, for which there was formerly but too good reason. They should be made and should be shown to be, first and foremost, not houses for detention, but hospitals for cure; and this can best be done by encouraging a more extensive knowledge of insanity in all its phases on the part of the general practitioner. Were this obtained, prejudices would be softened or effaced, patients would often be earlier submitted to proper treatment, a point vital for their chance of cure, and many more valuable members of the community saved to it, to their families, and to themselves.

"5, and finally. In claiming that even the interests of psychology and of superintendents would be benefited by the measure you instructed your delegate to urge, no more is stated than the facts in the case prove to be true. At Pittsburg it was alleged, privately and publicly, by more than one superintendent, that if the proposed union were effected, it would be the death-blow to their own Association. Such a result is not the object that yourselves have aimed to effect. Granting, however, that it should occur, would the dissolution referred to prove in reality detrimental to the best interests of medicine? That superintendents should desire to cultivate to a higher degree the brotherly feeling likely to exist among gentlemen engaged in a kindred occupation, where there is little or no possibility of their interfering with each other, is a very pleasant thing. Equally agreeable is it for one of their number each year to be able to exhibit his own establishment to his fellows, receive the encomiums certain in their generous rivalry to be deserved, and gain for himself the cumulative experience of so many kindly critics. But on the other hand, in medicine, the good of the greater number is sure, in the long run, to claim its own; and here in your midst are hungry souls, craving for the cases, countless almost as the sands on the seashore, of partial, incipient, or confirmed insanity, that as yet have never been at an asylum, or have been discharged as fit to remain at home, or incurable, more satisfying food regarding their rational causation, their treatment, or the prevention of the disease. These hospital superintendents have been set apart from their fellows, in part at least, because of their supposed illuminating power. Freed from the present self-imposed bushel of their own Association, then would their light shine so as to brighten the whole professional firmament.

"The officers of hospitals are compelled to rest, for a certain measure of their reputation, their influence, their power, upon yourselves outside; for it is by you that patients are advised to admission, their certificate of entrance signed, and the therapeutic judgment and conduct of those who take them in charge indorsed, in case, as so often happens, an appeal is made from themselves to a more public tribunal. It is you, moreover, who are to pronounce, year after year, and generation after generation, whether the same advance is made in the treatment of insanity that the divine mistress, whom we all serve, has a right to exact from her votaries. No branch of medicine can be dissevered from all others with safety to itself. Keeping aloof from the rest, it is easily distanced, and becomes effete. Or, if arrogantly claiming for itself exclusive rights, it by that act challenges an examination into the grounds of its assumption; if these prove lacking, then comes for it inevitably a fall from its high estate.

"Pregnant with practical and practicable idea, as is every relation of your profession to that great sickness, Insanity, worse than mortal, when incurable, there is one other point to which, in this connection, your delegate deems it well to draw your attention.

"It is well known that of all the cases interesting to medical jurists that enter our civil and criminal courts, those of insanity are the most perplexing. From the general initiatory question, In what does insanity consist? down to the special one of each particular occasion, Was or is this person insane? there is often exhibited a great and very conflicting diversity of sentiment; much of it undoubtedly necessary, because inherent in the questions themselves, and much of it capable of being removed. There is an equal variance of sentiment as to who shall, and who shall not be permitted to express his opinion as an expert, and who shall be entitled to credence. There exist, upon this point, wide extremes of opinion. Dr. Ray, for instance, in his "Medical Jurisprudence," and the able editor in chief of the American Journal of Insanity, Dr. Gray, of the Utica Asylum, as I have elsewhere shown, would confine this privilege or this ability to the few wise men who happen to hold positions at the head of an asylum. Sir Benjamin Brodie, on the other hand, a psychologist of no mean repute, extends it even to those beyond the ranks of the general profession, and declares that 'It is a great mistake to suppose that this is a question which can be determined only by medical practitioners. Any one,' he says, 'of plain, common sense, and having a fair knowledge of human nature, who will give it due consideration, is competent to form an opinion on it; and it belongs fully as much to those whose office it is to administer the law, as it does to the medical profession.' *

"A similar opinion has been expressed by one of your own body, the distinguished American editor of the Cyclopedia of Practical Medicine, the late Dr. Dunglison, of Philadelphia. Says this gentleman, 'In regard to the nature of the testimony relied upon in cases of insanity, and the mode of judging of the same, there is much room for animadversion. Too great weight appears to be given to medical testimony in such cases. It has always been the expressed conviction of the writer, that medical men are no better judges of the existence of mental alienation than well-informed and discriminating individuals not of the profession. The only advantage, at least, which they can be presumed to have, is from the constant habits of observation and discrimination, which the practical exercise of their profession requires. Yet, for no other reason than that they belong to the medical profession, inferior men, whose judgments on any other subject would be contemned, are often called upon to decide and establish the existence or nonexistence of a mental condition which demands the most careful and rigid scrutiny.'

"The same difference of opinion, shown above to obtain among medical men, exists also among the expounders of the law. Thus Wharton, justly celebrated alike for his treatise on Medical Jurisprudence and his several works upon Criminal Law, states that ' No juryman, if properly tender of his conscience and of public opinion, will base his verdict upon other evidence than that of those best able, from

* Mind and Matter; or, Physiological Inquiries, p. 105.

long training and close attention, to understand the features of the case. In some cases the difference between a scientific, or technical opinion, and that of a layman, is not so much in the results attained, as in the guarantee afforded by the superior attainments and more minute expertness of the man of science. The declaration of such a man is insured against the possibility of error to the full extent of the protection of science in its present stage of development. *Pro foro*, this degree of certainty is sufficient, because it is the highest attainable; but the same cannot be said of any other.'*

"Carried into court, however, it is found that the rulings upon this point have been diametrically opposed to each other. In New York, the Court of Appeals has decided, though with a strong dissenting sentiment, that none but professional witnesses are competent to testify on the subject of insanity (Dewitt *v.* Barley & Schoonmaker, 5 Selden, 371), while the Supreme Court of the same State admits the opinions of laymen (Culver *v.* Haslem, 7 Barb., 314). In Pennsylvania the point has been settled in favor of admitting the testimony of non-professional witnesses (Rambler *v.* Tryan, 7 Serg. & Rawle, 90; Wogan *v.* Small, 11 Serg. & Rawle, 141). In Connecticut, decisions have been of a similar character (Grant *v.* Thompson, 4 Conn., 203). In Indiana, provided the facts are stated upon which his opinions are founded, an unprofessional witness may express his opinion regarding the existence of insanity (Doe *v.* Reagan, 5 Black., 217). The same is true in Tennessee, North Carolina, and Ohio (Gibson *v.* Gibson, 9 Yerger, 329; Clary *v.* Clary, 2 Iredell's Law Rep., 78; The State *v.* Clark, 12 Ohio, 483); and in Vermont also (Lester *v.* Pittsford, 7 Verm., 158; Morse *v.* Crawford, 19 Id., 499).

"In view of these facts, either of the above-mentioned extreme decisions being disadvantageous to the mass of your profession, as refusing to you, on the one hand, competence to express any opinion in cases which you may

---

* Medical Jurisprudence, § 91.

perhaps have watched closely for years, and extending, on the other, equal rights and privileges with yourselves, in purely professional matters, to the most unprofessional persons, it is not improper to urge upon you action, which, if taken, will also serve to render the measure you have thus far in vain proposed effective. The action advised is as follows: to render the study of medical jurisprudence, in which insanity holds so important a place, more prominent at our medical schools than it has ever yet been.

"Of the propriety of such a step, few of our teachers have ever doubted. It has more than once been urged upon this Association, in the valuable reports upon the subject presented to you by Drs. Coventry, of Utica, and Reese, of New York City. Now that the Association has again risen, with more than youthful vigor, from the ashes of the past, it should be no vain hope that the wise suggestions made to you nearly ten years since may be carried into effect. Long ago it was the complaint of that Nestor of American psychological writers, Dr. Pliny Earle, that this 'subject of insanity does not enter into the programme of lectures in any of our leading medical schools. It is safe, perhaps, to assert,' he says, 'that not one in ten of the graduates of those schools has ever read a treatise upon mental disorders.' 'Indeed,' says one of your reporters to whom I have referred, 'the department of medical jurisprudence itself is either wholly ignored in the curriculum of our universities and colleges, or merely appended to some other chair or chairs, by way of formal recognition, and this, for the most part, *stat nominis umbra*.' And again: 'The demands of our civil and criminal courts all over the land, for competent and intelligent medical testimony, must be met by raising up an army of experts in every department of medical jurisprudence, and especially on this important topic of mental aberration. Else the ignorance of too many physicians, displayed before the courts and juries, may lead to the undervaluation, if not the rejection, of medical evidence in all such cases.'*

---

* Report on Moral Insanity in its Relations to Medical Jurisprudence Transactions of the American Medical Association, 1858.

"Attempts have been made, it is true, to initiate a change, but, at best, they have been but feeble and imperfect. At Harvard University the special subject of insanity is lectured upon by Dr. Tyler, and, at Pittsfield, Dr. Earle was called not long since to a similar duty, until forbidden to pursue the subject by the trustees of his asylum, upon the ground that it took him from the more legitimate offices of his position as superintendent. As yet the evil upon which he himself so forcibly commented remains unchanged. In but a few of our schools, whether of medicine or of law, is the important subject of medical jurisprudence viewed with a tithe of the interest it deserves; in others, if touched upon at all, it is only as an appendage, like a caudal fin, as has well been said by one of its own professors, to some other chair, improperly considered as of more importance. This indifference has, no doubt, in part been owing to the lack of competent instructors, who, to be properly fitted for their task, should themselves be masters alike of medicine and of the law. Teachers, however, would have been long since forthcoming, had the colleges called for them. As a strong proof of the argument now made, let your delegate state that in a letter lately received from that justly eminent and very competent instructor, Dr. John Ordronaux, of New York, the fact is mentioned that this gentleman now lectures upon medical jurisprudence in no less than five professional schools, to wit, two law and three medical; and these, it is perhaps not too much to say, are almost the only instances in which this science is as yet at all properly taught in this country.

"There is no class of experts against whom the bolts of legal practitioners, alike counsel and judges, have been so unsparingly hurled, as against those claiming to speak as medical jurists. Particularly does this occur in cases of insanity; and in none has so much real damage been done to the profession, not always, either, with entire injustice. The exigencies of the case, aggressive and defensive, have been so great, that the subject has lately been taken in hand, with a view to decided action, by one of the highest courts of professional appeal in the country, the American Academy of Arts and Sciences, the whole matter having been under examination by a committee, of which the Chief Justice of Massachusetts was chairman, and of which your delegate has had the honor to be a member. As parties deeply interested in any movement that can better yourselves and advance the interests of the profession, it lies with you to assist in this work.

"Your delegate would therefore, while trespassing no longer upon your patience by argument, offer for adoption two mutually dependent resolutions, the second of them being based, he would recall to your recollection, upon action taken at your last meeting, at the suggestion of Dr. Edward Jarvis, the well-known statistical psychologist, in accordance with which a Section of Psychological Medicine, intended more particularly for the reception of the superintendents, was organized by this Association. It is a source of great satisfaction that yesterday, for the first time, the new section was formally convened. The high character of the half dozen gentlemen, all of them connected with the specialty of insanity, who took part in its deliberations, and the important work that they accomplished, which was no less than assigning a special scientific investigation to the most celebrated member of their fraternity, Dr. Isaac Ray, are an earnest that your interests in this direction will not be allowed to languish. More is required, however, than has thus far been effected. It is necessary that the great body of superintendents should convene at the same time and place with yourselves, and thus, without in reality interfering with their enjoyment and their consentaneousness of action, that their interests should become more clearly identified with your own.

"The resolutions now offered are the following; for their passage still additional arguments would have been presented, had such seemed necessary: —

"1. *Resolved*, That the Association recommend to the several medical and law schools of the country the establishment of an independent chair of medical jurisprudence, to be filled, if possible, by teachers who have studied both law and medicine; attendance upon one full course of lectures from whom shall be deemed necessary before the medical degree is conferred.

"2. *Resolved*, That while this Association regrets that the Association of Superintendents of American Asylums for the Insane has not yet thought fit to unite itself more closely with the representative body of American physicians, it still is of opinion that such union is for their mutual and reciprocal advantage, and that it ought to be effected without further delay.

"All of which is respectfully submitted."

The resolutions above presented were unanimously adopted by the Association.

As the present leaf of this book is passing through the press, I have received a most interesting commentary upon its last few pages. At the annual meeting for the present year (1870) of the Association of Medical Superintendents of American Asylums for the Insane, the official report[*] of which has just reached me, these gentlemen were assured by the delegate from the American Medical Association, Dr. John L. Atlee, of Pennsylvania, that their union with the General Association would be impolitic, both for themselves and the profession at large. "We have enough to do," said Dr. Atlee, "in devoting our time to the other departments of medicine, without including the subject of insanity," — a remark as applicable to all other classes of disease whatso-

[*] American Journal of Insanity, October, 1870, p. 129.

ever. Under these circumstances, Dr. Atlee was, of course, congratulated by the superintendents for his alleged good sense, and his remarks will, doubtless, be still further lauded by Dr. Tyler, of the Somerville Asylum, in his report upon the subject, that his recent illness has delayed until next year.

Notwithstanding all this, I still submit that the meetings of the two Associations, so long as they shall remain distinct, should at least be held at the same place each year, and nearly simultaneously, the one immediately preceding or following the other. In the immediate vicinity of all our large cities there are now insane asylums, to visit which it is naturally so pleasant to superintendents.

It must not be forgotten, moreover, that Dr. Atlee is, and has long been, a manager of one of the Pennsylvania State Asylums, and that, as he is therefore necessarily identified in feeling, as he has indeed shown himself to be, with the members of the specialty, his opinion upon the question referred to must be received with a good deal of hesitancy.

The remarks made at the same meeting, upon the relations of uterine disease to insanity, by Dr. James P. White, of Buffalo, also a manager of a State Asylum, and President of its Board, are in every way to be admired. Professor White, like Dr. Atlee, is well known as one of the best gynæcologists in the country; and from the efforts he has made, through the

American Medical Association, to procure the establishment of professorships of mental disease at all our medical colleges, his opinions cannot but have great weight with those in charge of asylums.

Thus it will be seen that there are signs that the great reform in the treatment of the female insane, for which we have so long been laboring, will, at no distant day, become accomplished.

Medicine & Society In America

An Arno Press/New York Times Collection

Alcott, William A. **The Physiology of Marriage.** 1866. New Introduction by Charles E. Rosenberg.

Beard, George M. **American Nervousness:** Its Causes and Consequences. 1881. New Introduction by Charles E. Rosenberg.

Beard, George M. **Sexual Neurasthenia.** 5th edition. 1898.

Beecher, Catharine E. **Letters to the People on Health and Happiness.** 1855.

Blackwell, Elizabeth. **Essays in Medical Sociology.** 1902. Two volumes in one.

Blanton, Wyndham B. **Medicine in Virginia in the Seventeenth Century.** 1930.

Bowditch, Henry I. **Public Hygiene in America.** 1877.

Bowditch, N[athaniel] I. **A History of the Massachusetts General Hospital:** To August 5, 1851. 2nd edition. 1872.

Brill, A. A. **Psychanalysis:** Its Theories and Practical Application. 1913.

Cabot, Richard C. **Social Work:** Essays on the Meeting-Ground of Doctor and Social Worker. 1919.

Cathell, D. W. **The Physician Himself and What He Should Add to His Scientific Acquirements.** 2nd edition. 1882. New Introduction by Charles E. Rosenberg.

The Cholera Bulletin. Conducted by an Association of Physicians. Vol. I: Nos. 1–24. 1832. All published. New Introduction by Charles E. Rosenberg.

Clarke, Edward H. **Sex in Education;** or, A Fair Chance for the Girls. 1873.

Committee on the Costs of Medical Care. **Medical Care for the American People:** The Final Report of The Committee on the Costs of Medical Care, No. 28. [1932].

Currie, William. **An Historical Account of the Climates and Diseases of the United States of America.** 1792.

Davenport, Charles Benedict. **Heredity in Relation to Eugenics.** 1911. New Introduction by Charles E. Rosenberg.

Davis, Michael M. **Paying Your Sickness Bills.** 1931.

Disease and Society in Provincial Massachusetts: Collected Accounts, 1736–1939. 1972.

Earle, Pliny. **The Curability of Insanity:** A Series of Studies. 1887.

Falk, I. S., C. Rufus Rorem, and Martha D. Ring. **The Costs of Medical Care:** A Summary of Investigations on The Economic Aspects of the Prevention and Care of Illness, No. 27. 1933.

Faust, Bernhard C. **Catechism of Health:** For the Use of Schools, and for Domestic Instruction. 1794.

Flexner, Abraham. **Medical Education in the United States and Canada:** A Report to The Carnegie Foundation for the Advancement of Teaching, Bulletin Number Four. 1910.

Gross, Samuel D. **Autobiography of Samuel D. Gross, M.D.**, with Sketches of His Contemporaries. Two volumes. 1887.

Hooker, Worthington. **Physician and Patient**; or, A Practical View of the Mutual Duties, Relations and Interests of the Medical Profession and the Community. 1849.

Howe, S. G. **On the Causes of Idiocy.** 1858.

Jackson, James. **A Memoir of James Jackson, Jr., M.D.** 1835.

Jennings, Samuel K. **The Married Lady's Companion, or Poor Man's Friend.** 2nd edition. 1808.

The Maternal Physician; a Treatise on the Nurture and Management of Infants, from the Birth until Two Years Old. 2nd edition. 1818. New Introduction by Charles E. Rosenberg.

Mathews, Joseph McDowell. **How to Succeed in the Practice of Medicine.** 1905.

McCready, Benjamin W. **On the Influences of Trades, Professions, and Occupations in the United States, in the Production of Disease.** 1943.

Mitchell, S. Weir. **Doctor and Patient.** 1888.

Nichols, T[homas] L. **Esoteric Anthropology: The Mysteries of Man.** [1853].

Origins of Public Health in America: Selected Essays, 1820–1855. 1972.

Osler, Sir William. **The Evolution of Modern Medicine.** 1922.

The Physician and Child-Rearing: Two Guides, 1809–1894. 1972.

Rosen, George. **The Specialization of Medicine:** with Particular Reference to Ophthalmology. 1944.

Royce, Samuel. **Deterioration and Race Education.** 1878.

Rush, Benjamin. **Medical Inquiries and Observations.** Four volumes in two. 4th edition. 1815.

Shattuck, Lemuel, Nathaniel P. Banks, Jr., and Jehiel Abbott. **Report of a General Plan for the Promotion of Public and Personal Health.** Massachusetts Sanitary Commission. 1850.

Smith, Stephen. **Doctor in Medicine** and Other Papers on Professional Subjects. 1872.

Still, Andrew T. **Autobiography of Andrew T. Still,** with a History of the Discovery and Development of the Science of Osteopathy. 1897.

Storer, Horatio Robinson. **The Causation, Course, and Treatment of Reflex Insanity in Women.** 1871.

Sydenstricker, Edgar. **Health and Environment.** 1933.

Thomson, Samuel. **A Narrative, of the Life and Medical Discoveries of Samuel Thomson.** 1822.

Ticknor, Caleb. **The Philosophy of Living;** or, The Way to Enjoy Life and Its Comforts. 1836.

U.S. Sanitary Commission. **The Sanitary Commission of the United States Army:** A Succinct Narrative of Its Works and Purposes. 1864.

White, William A. **The Principles of Mental Hygiene.** 1917.

NO LONGER THE PROPERTY
OF THE
UNIVERSITY OF R.I. LIBRARY